PREGNANCY
BLUES

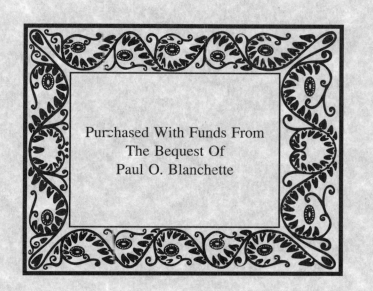

PREGNANCY BLUES

What Every Woman
Needs to Know About
Depression During Pregnancy

SHAILA KULKARNI MISRI, M.D., F.R.C.P.C.

DELACORTE PRESS

PREGNANCY BLUES
A Delacorte Press Book / September 2005

Published by Bantam Dell
A Division of Random House, Inc.
New York, New York

Book design by Helene Berinsky

Delacorte Press is a registered trademark of Random House, Inc.,
and the colophon is a trademark of Random House, Inc.

Library of Congress Cataloging in Publication Data
Misri, Shaila.
Pregnancy blues : what every women needs to know about
depression during pregnancy / Shaila Kulkarni Misri.
p.   cm.
Includes bibliographical references and index.
ISBN 0-385-33866-X
1. Postpartum depression. 2. Postpartum depression—Treatment.
3. Pregnancy—Psychological aspects. 4. Depression in women.
5. Mental illness in pregnancy. I. Title.
RG852.M57 2005
618.7'6—dc22   2005045557

Printed in the United States of America
Published simultaneously in Canada

www.bantamdell.com

BVG   10   9   8   7   6   5   4   3   2   1

This book is for informational purposes only. It is not intended as a diagnostic tool or prescription manual, or to replace the advice and care of a qualified medical doctor. Although every effort has been made to provide the most up-to-date information, the medical science in this field and information about depression and pharmacological treatments is rapidly changing. Furthermore, the medical concerns of a woman's pregnancy and mental health are unique to each patient and require individual attention and care. Accordingly, we strongly recommend that you consult with your doctor before acting on any of the information imparted in this book.

To Nate and Nick—my pride and joy

To Babi—my soulmate

To Mandakini—my guide

To Shivrao—my inspiration

To Bhau and Balu—the proud Kulkarnis

ACKNOWLEDGMENTS

Drs. Diana Carter, Deirdre Ryan, Maria Corral, Jackie Hui, Shimi Kang, and nurse clinician Barb Komar—had it not been for all of you, who helped carry the burden of patients when I took time off to write this book, I most certainly could not have achieved my goal. I want to express my gratitude for your unfailing support and patience. I also want to thank the other members of the Reproductive Mental Health Program for your ongoing encouragement.

Amy O'Conner, it was you who inspired me to write another book.

Dorian Karchmar, my literary agent, you stood by me through the difficult as well as the good times and never gave up on me. Your enthusiasm is matched by your professionalism. You have been more than an advisor and a negotiator; you were determined to see this book in print, for which I thank you from the bottom of my heart.

Judy Kern, you were instrumental in making this book a reality every step of the way, from start to finish. Without your invaluable contribution, input, conceptual framework, and editing, this book would not have taken the shape or form it has today. Your patient revisions and expertise in writing are unparalleled. It has been a pleasure to work on this book with you. No words can thank you enough.

Danielle Perez, my editor at Bantam Dell, I valued your critical evaluation of the manuscript and always-helpful comments. I also want to express my thanks for your confidence in my work, which has enabled me to share my knowledge with the rest of the world.

Lisa Milis, you saw the book at its conception, and I'm just sorry that you couldn't be there for its birth! Your commitment, determination, and devotion to this project have been remarkable, and I will always remain grateful for all that you have done. Kristin Kendrick, thank you for jumping in whenever I needed you; you are never afraid to take on a new challenge. Ruth Little, thank you for all of your help as well.

Lloyd Cain, I'm indebted to you for your speedy transcription skills and your punctual delivery. You have been dependable and simply terrific. Thank you, Jean MacLaren, for pitching in whenever I needed you. Dean Giustini, I thank you for finding the time to help me with the library search despite your busy schedule.

Liezel and Christine, you two put up with my ever-changing schedule; without your understanding and unlimited tolerance, I could not have gone through this long, arduous process.

As always, Bushan, my husband, your belief in me and your confidence in my writing outweighed my own. Nathaniel and Nick, my two priceless children, you both were wonderful; never complaining, never disturbing me while I was working away at the book during your summer vacation. My brothers, Dilip and Deepak Kulkarni—I know you are proud of my work. And, although you are thousands of miles away, I thank you, Mom, for being there for me in spirit. I also want to recognize my late father, whose power with written words motivated me to write; thank you, Dad.

Finally, without you, my patients, this book would never have become a reality. I am honored that you trusted me and shared your lives with me. I remain beholden.

And if I have forgotten to mention anyone's name, I apologize and assure you that I am grateful for your help.

CONTENTS

PREGNANCY BLUES

INTRODUCTION

When I started medical school in my native India in the mid-1960s, becoming a psychiatrist hadn't even entered my mind. In fact, several members of my family were either obstetricians or surgeons, and as a child, I'd always dreamed of becoming an obstetrician myself.

Beginning at the age of sixteen, I spent my summers with an uncle who was the only surgeon and obstetrician in the town where he lived and who, knowing of my interest in medicine, gave me the opportunity to put on a pair of surgical gloves and act as his assistant. Sometimes I was so distressed by the pained cries of the women in labor that I actually thought I might faint. But even so, I knew that somehow, in some capacity, I would continue to be involved in the field of obstetrics.

As time went on and I completed one year of training in obstetrics and gynecology in Europe, I found that the psychological aspects of pregnancy and childbirth were as intriguing as the physiological. And so, when I came to Canada in the mid-1970s, I applied for residencies in both obstetrics and psychiatry. As luck (or fate) would have it, the department of psychiatry was the first to accept me, with the department of obstetrics following six months later. So I started my psychiatric residency fully intent on returning, in time, to my first love: obstetrics. As it turned out, I was both right and wrong!

My interest in pregnant and postpartum women really peaked in the last year of my psychiatric training when my professor, Dr. Ralph Schulman, would send me over to see these "pregnant ladies" (as he referred to them) and report back to him on their issues and problems. What soon became blatantly clear was, first of all, that their problems weren't being taken very seriously and, second, that many of them did not improve after they gave birth but continued to have severe psychiatric illnesses that none of us, including myself, was adequately trained to address. Finding a way to help those women became my personal mission.

My psychiatric residency completed, I approached the head of the department of obstetrics about opening a psychiatric clinic at the maternity hospital. I started with a small, borrowed office in the outpatient department, and within a year the waiting list had outgrown even my wildest expectations. Today that small "temporary" space has grown into the Reproductive Mental Health Program, with a staff of eight women psychiatrists, three counseling psychologists, three clinical nurse specialists, four clinical clerks, and four research assistants. We see approximately two to three thousand women a year on an outpatient basis as well as counsel pregnant and postpartum patients in Women's Hospital and St. Paul's Hospital. We provide education and therapy both in groups and one-on-one, conduct research, and train medical and nursing students, as well as trainees, from other disciplines.

Twenty years ago, when the program was in its infancy, most of our patients were referred because they were suffering postpartum depression. Today, however, that pattern has changed, and far more of the women we see are dealing with depression during pregnancy. Although postpartum depression is now accepted as a unique illness with diagnostic criteria included in the *Diagnostic and Statistical Manual of Psychiatric Disorders*, and has recently been the subject of unprecedented focus as the result of a few tragic cases that received international attention, pregnancy-related depression all too often remains hidden in plain sight. My hope for this book is to change that.

Since the publication of *What to Expect When You're Expecting* almost twenty years ago, more than ten million women have learned to be alert and tuned in to even the slightest physiological change they are likely to experience during pregnancy. Far fewer women, however, have any idea how to recognize depression when it strikes or even realize that being pregnant may put them at risk for becoming depressed. Many, in fact, still believe not only that pregnancy will protect them from depression but also that it, in and of itself, can actually bring about relief.

My purpose here is not to frighten women into fearing that if they become pregnant they will become depressed. On the contrary, for the great majority of women pregnancy is indeed a period of joyous anticipation. But I do want to make it clear that for women who are depressed, pregnancy is not a cure; for those who have experienced bouts of depression in the past, it may trigger a relapse; and for some, pregnancy will act as a trigger for depression.

Although I no longer hear women crying out in labor on a daily basis (and it's been years since I thought I would faint), I now hear and bear witness to their psychic pain, and to me, those cries—although often silent—sound louder and more anguished.

In the pages that follow, I'll be exploring the psychosocial and biological factors that can come together during pregnancy to create a climate in which depression thrives. I'll be explaining how to recognize its symptoms and why it is so important to seek help. Most important of all, I'll address all the issues surrounding the ongoing controversy about whether or not to take psychiatric medications during pregnancy and postpartum.

Having worked with and medicated both pregnant and postpartum depressed women for more than a quarter of a century, having read all the available research, and having been personally involved in significant groundbreaking studies, I can state with utmost confidence that allowing depression to go untreated is far more dangerous to both the mother and her baby than taking medication that is properly prescribed and monitored or considering other forms of therapies. But I also understand that this is an area that is bound to generate a great deal of fear, in large part because it has for so long been surrounded by silence and secrecy. I am a firm believer in the power to be gained through education and knowledge, and my purpose here is to empower women to become fully enlightened partners in their own psychiatric care.

PART

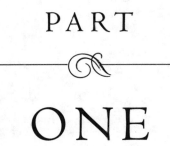

ONE

I

Great Expectations

CULTURAL MYTHS, CUSTOMS, AMBIGUITIES,
AND MISCONCEPTIONS OF WOMANHOOD,
PREGNANCY, AND MOTHERHOOD

If some enterprising salesperson were to create a pregnant woman's coloring book aimed at the North American market, it would surely come packaged with a box containing nothing but pastel crayons with names like Blissful Blue, Perfect Pink, and Mother's Mauve. No Black Cloud, Blue Funk, or Red Rage in that crayon box! And the mothers outlined in the book for coloring would all be smiling serenely, gazing lovingly into the eyes of their partner—an equally blissed-out expectant father—and, of course, looking nothing less than beautiful.

If that sounds like the Hollywood image of pregnancy, it is certainly the one that's been sold to Western women, and that Western culture has naively bought in to. For the majority of women, it is probably even a fair approximation of the truth. It is not, however, the image of pregnancy that I see every day. And if we look a little more closely at the myths and mixed messages that have historically surrounded fertility, family, and femininity not only in our society but in cultures throughout the world, we can see that—as is so often the case with the images Hollywood has for sale—this is one that may have been meant for viewing through rose-colored glasses.

To begin close to home, let's take a quick look back at the history of our own North American culture as it has grown from a mainly agrarian to a mainly technological society. In times past, when we tilled fields, worked the land, and subsisted mainly on what a single family could produce for both sale and sustenance, children were important assets. As farmers, ranchers, or even local shopkeepers, we needed those extra hands to work alongside us and help to support us. Fertility and motherhood were, therefore, valued as well, and a woman's primary role, aside from taking care of the family homestead, was to produce and nurture children. "Mother" was a prized and universally recognized job title.

I know that for many modern women, reading about the difficult and often isolated lives of those pioneer and farm wives will immediately bring to mind the now-classic advertising slogan "You've come a long way, baby!" And indeed we have. But that also begs the question "Where have we arrived?" In many ways, of course, the lives of twenty-first-century women are dramatically better. And it's certainly true that, from a medical perspective, obstetrical care is better and more universally available than ever before. But what about the lives of mothers, and even the value we put on motherhood itself?

For the majority of Western women today, motherhood, rather than being a primary function, has become no more than an add-on. Even those of us who truly yearn for children, who unwaveringly wish for the chance to be mothers, are unlikely either to perceive motherhood as our only goal or to have the luxury of enjoying it as our only job title.

In a technologically driven society, pregnancy is too often perceived as an interruption of or an addition to other, more valued activities. At best, we are ambivalent about where pregnancy and motherhood belong on our list of priorities. "Stay-at-home mom" and "mommy track" are terms that have entered our vocabulary with a kind of stigma attached. Women who choose (and have the luxury of choosing) to opt out of the job market or limit their career path in order to spend more time with their children are often marginalized by and isolated from their working peers. Those who choose to pursue both career and motherhood, on the other hand, are often made to explain or justify their choice to those who believe they "should" stay at home. And for the majority of women who simply do not have a choice, pregnancy and motherhood present financial as well as logistical burdens that can be overwhelming.

In fact, throughout history and across cultural boundaries, woman's unique ability to bear children has put her in the position of being both worshiped and feared; it has been her source of power and her burden, a blessing and a curse. Religion and mythology, which brim not only with female fertility figures such as the Buddhist Kwan Yin, the Hindu Lakshmi, and the Egyptian Isis but also with seductresses such as Lilith and Diana, reflect this dichotomy. Even the Virgin Mary, the most universally recognized mother figure of them all, is not only blessed to be the mother of the Christ, worshiped as the intermediary between the human and the divine, but also born to bear the burden of becoming the Mater Dolorosa, the mother who weeps for the loss of her only child and the sins of humanity.

This ambiguity or dual nature inherent in the concept of "womanhood" is also reflected in religious and cultural issues related to women's bodily functions. The Orthodox Jewish community, for example, considers a menstruating woman unclean. She is forbidden to have sexual relations with her husband and required, when her period is over, to immerse herself in a ritual bath not once but three times to ensure that any lingering impurities are washed away. Here we can see the duality that exists between woman as the bearer of children and woman as temptress: if she is menstruating, she cannot become pregnant, her potential for motherhood is temporarily negated, and so for her husband to have sexual relations with her during this time would be to give in to her powers of seduction—to be, in a sense, defiled by her.

Similarly, in traditional Hindu culture, women were considered both inferior to men and, at the same time, capable of seducing them away from ascetic contemplation and spiritual purity. Only through motherhood did they cement and ensure their power base through their almost total influence over their children and the household.

In these and other traditional cultures, motherhood not only endows women with a kind of retrofitted purity but also initiates them into a special company of women. In many communities throughout Asia, Africa, and South America women generally give birth surrounded by other women, and following the delivery there is a traditional period of confinement during which both mother and child are tended and nurtured by women.

In many cultures, there is a special birthing place set aside, which only women can enter, and very often—such as among the women of Yemen, the Gbaya of Congo, or the Seri Indians of Mexico—that can mean as many as fifteen female friends, neighbors, and family members in addition to the midwife present to witness the birth. Even in Elizabethan England, men were banned from the birthing chamber while female friends, relatives, and neighbors, known as "gossips," were invited to attend. Some, in fact, might spend days or even weeks after the birth attending the mother in her room.

This "lying-in" period is still practiced in many cultures. In Cuba, for example, the new mother and her infant remain inside the home for forty-one days, during which time women from the family and the community are responsible for taking care of them. In India women are not expected to return to their normal household chores for more than a month. Bedouin women stay home for forty days, are not allowed to cook or do housework, and are expected to rest and eat well. In China the traditional period of confinement is one month, in Malaysia it is forty-four days, and among the Igbo people of southeastern Nigeria it is one lunar month, during which time the mother is relieved of all chores, given special foods, and nursed by her own mother or an older sister.

Although these are certainly periods set aside for mother and baby to bond (in most instances the infant actually remains in bed with the mother and can nurse at will) and for the mother to recover, they also mark another rite of passage—from girlhood to womanhood or, seen from another perspective, from seductress to saint. It should be pointed out, in fact, that in at least some cultures, the period of confinement is also considered a time of repurification following the "pollution" of childbirth.

But how do such practices relate to pregnancy and motherhood in our own culture? Again, I think it is enlightening to examine this question from more than one perspective.

On one hand, although the vast majority of modern Western women deliver their babies in far more sterile conditions, we also miss out on the benefits to be derived from the closeness and care of other women. For the most part, we give birth surrounded not by those who are necessarily closest and most caring but by paid professionals and coldly beeping machinery. Our "lying-in" period in the hospital is barely twenty-four hours, after which we are sent home to cope as best we can. We might have a mother who is both able and willing to help out, but even if we are so lucky, her stay generally lasts no more than a week or two. We might be granted maternity leave by our employer, but we generally spend that time in relative isolation. Our period of transition is spent not being coddled and cared for but in 24/7 on-the-job training. We are expected either to know instinctively how to mother or to learn the ropes by reading books as we muddle along. At the same time, we are undergoing another important—and not necessarily happy—transition with relation to our own sense of self.

It's hard, when we're usually exhausted, still overweight, and often bedraggled, wearing a nursing bra or wiping formula from our clothing, to remember who we were just nine months before. In fact, many of us are undergoing our own personal reassessment and seeing ourselves as no longer seductive, if not quite as saints (although from time to time we might consider ourselves deserving of sainthood).

The messages we receive from the media may suggest that we ought to be self-confidently sexual when pregnant—like Brooke Shields on the cover of *Vogue* or Demi Moore, nude and in full body paint, adorning *Vanity Fair*. Then, having given birth, we ought to be "ready for our close-up," as coiffed and composed as Gwyneth Paltrow, as skinny as Sarah Jessica Parker, as coolly elegant as Catherine Zeta-Jones. But do these images really make us feel better about ourselves, or do they just remind us that we are somehow not living up to expectations? Perhaps we'd be better off if, like women in earlier times and more traditional cultures, we had a clearer picture of our new role and place in the world. We'd certainly be better off if motherhood, in and of itself, were looked upon with the kind of dignity and respect it is shown in other cultures.

But then again, is this not just one more of the mixed messages women constantly receive about their value as bearers of children? Even in societies where the mother's role is recognized as intrinsically worthy of respect, girl children—the future childbearers and mothers, it should be pointed out—are afforded second-class status. In some parts of India a boy baby is still welcomed as a future helper and contributor to the family's wealth, while a girl, assuming she is even allowed to survive and remain in her family of birth, is looked upon as a burden and an additional drain on the family's income. And in China the government-mandated one-child population-control policy has led to a precipitous decline in the ratio of girl to boy babies. Indeed, in that country, where for centuries male offspring have represented continuity of lineage and financial support, the abortion or infanticide of girls has created a situation where there will soon not be enough young women to produce the prized male heirs of the future. And the legacy of this centuries-old gender bias is still seen, at least ceremonially, even in Great Britain, where the birth of a male heir to the throne is greeted with a 101-gun salute while a female heir rates no more than 21.

We need to ask ourselves, then, what emotional and psychological effect all these conflicting images of femininity, myths of power, and messages of value (or lack thereof) might have on women, whose sole unique, biologically endowed capability is to bear and nurture children. Yes, of course, we want to think of conceiving and bringing a new life into the world as an occasion for joyous celebration—and for the majority of women, it is.

For a significant minority, however, who may have subliminally internalized the ambiguities inherent in the way society views motherhood, who may themselves be unconsciously ambivalent about the role they are about to take on, or who may become suddenly and glaringly aware of the life-changing transition they are about to undertake, pregnancy and childbirth can—and do—create the perfect emotional and biological climate for the onset of negative thoughts and feelings that lead to anxiety and even major depression. In the pages that follow we'll be looking at the many ways in which societal pressures and expectations, internal stress, and women's unique biology may come together to color a pregnancy in shades of gray and black.

I believe it's time to take off those rose-colored glasses and look at a picture of pregnancy that may not be as pretty as the one that's been painted by the media but which is, for too many women, sadly more realistic. Until we are willing to do that, we are unwittingly sentencing these women to continue hiding in plain sight, unable or unwilling to admit, perhaps even to themselves, that their experience of pregnancy is not what they've been taught to expect, and that what appears to be so joyful for others is for them a time of sadness, fear, and confusion. These women need to know that it doesn't have to be that way, that there is help, and that they cannot and should not be embarrassed or afraid to get the help they need. Indeed, this book is filled with the stories of women who *have* come out of hiding and who have, as a result, turned a potentially devastating experience into one that not only was manageable but also ultimately did bring them the joy of bonding with a happy, healthy baby.

2

Depression

THE FEMALE PLAGUE

B efore we discuss how and why depression is likely to affect women both during pregnancy and in the postpartum period, it's important to understand that, in general, women are statistically more likely than men to experience a major depression at some point in their lives, and particularly during their reproductive years. A recent article in a prominent medical journal referred to depression as a modern version of the bubonic plague. Unlike the plague, depression is not a contagious disease, and yet it plagues a staggering number of people, the majority of whom are women.

The statistics alone are overwhelming. The World Health Organization has determined that depression affects approximately fifty million people throughout the world. More than 15 percent of the population is afflicted with this illness and a large proportion with its associated disabilities.

Major depression, as defined by the *Diagnostic and Statistical Manual of Mental Disorders (DSM-IV-TR)* of the American Psychiatric Association, is the most common of all the psychiatric disorders; with the exception of high blood pressure, it is the condition most commonly encountered by family physicians. Depression is the cause of more functional impairment and poorer quality of life than diabetes, heart disease, or high blood pressure. Is it surprising, then that depression has a worse prognosis than any medical disorder except advanced coronary artery disease? In fact, 15 percent of people diagnosed with depression ultimately commit suicide.

For women in particular, the statistics are even more devastating. The prevalence of depression in women is about 20 percent as opposed to 10 percent in men, according to the National Comorbidity Survey. In other words, women are twice as likely as men to suffer from depression, and in the United States specifically the lifetime rate of risk for depression is 1.7 to 2.4 times greater for women. In 1990 the World Health Organization found it to be the leading cause of disability in women of childbearing years.

Medicine has made great strides in recent years, discovering the causes of, curing, and even wiping out various diseases, but despite the shocking numbers recorded for depression, until 2002 the U.S. Preventive Services Task Force and the Agency for Healthcare Research and Quality didn't even recommend screening for depression because its symptoms were so amorphous and its incidence did not seem sufficient to warrant the outlay of public funds.

The symptoms of major depression are defined by *DSM-IV-TR* as follows:

Psychological symptoms	Physical symptoms
• Depressed mood most of the day nearly every day	• Sleep disturbance (insomnia or hypersomnia)
• Reduction of interest and/or pleasure in activities, including sex	• Appetite/weight changes • Attention/concentration difficulties
• Feelings of guilt, hopelessness, and worthlessness	• Decreased energy or unexplained fatigue
• Suicidal thoughts	• Psychomotor disturbances

A. For the diagnosis of major depression, five or more of the above symptoms must be present during the same two-week period,

and represent a change from previous functioning. At least one
of the symptoms must be either depressed mood or loss of
interest or pleasure.

B. The symptoms do not meet criteria for a mixed episode.

C. The symptoms cause significant distress or impairment in
social and/or occupational functioning.

D. The symptoms are not due to substance use or a medical
condition.

E. The symptoms are not caused by the loss of a loved one, and
persist for two months.

Adapted from the American Psychiatric Association. *Diagnostic and Statistical
Manual of Mental Disorders, 4th ed., Text Revision (DSM-IV-TR)* (Washington, D.C.:
American Psychiatric Association, 2000).

Depression Is Insidious

Amorphous or nebulous as its symptoms may be, at least at the outset,
depression is also insidious. If you break a bone or scald yourself with
boiling water, there is immediate acute pain, and the source of that pain
is instantly apparent. Depression, however, doesn't present itself with
such obvious and immediate symptoms. Rather, the mental and physical changes it causes creep up gradually, sometimes over a period of
years, eating away at and eroding one's quality of life, and very often the
person who is suffering is the last to recognize what's happening to
him—or more likely, her.

When she came to see me, Nora was twenty-three years old and contemplating her first pregnancy. Her mother, a high school teacher, was
there to support her on this visit. A lovely green-eyed, raven-haired
young woman, Nora remembered having felt "blue" and missing school
as far back as when she was just fourteen years old. Her mother, who
was an intelligent and rational woman who had modeled the value of

education through her work, simply couldn't understand why *her* daughter, of all people, wouldn't want to go to school. Of course, she had tried to reason with Nora (reason, after all, was the only way Nora's mother knew to approach problem solving), and after that, Nora did go to school, but she spent her days roaming the halls and visiting with friends, not attending classes. Her mother was shocked and felt completely helpless when, at the end of the year, the principal informed her that Nora was being left back because she'd missed so many classes.

At that point, the only way Nora's mother was able to cope with the situation was not to deal with it at all, so she shut herself off from her daughter completely. And Nora's father, a salesman who spent much of his time on the road, remained totally clueless about what was going on at home.

When school began again the following fall, Nora didn't even have the energy or wherewithal to *pretend* she was going to class. She spent most of her days in bed sleeping and found it difficult to complete even the simplest of tasks. Not until then did Nora's aunt insist to her parents that this was clearly not normal behavior for a fourteen-year-old girl and that Nora desperately needed professional help.

What's particularly sad to me about Nora's story is the fact that her condition had to deteriorate to the point where she was virtually nonfunctional before anyone intervened. If her pain had been physical rather than emotional, her mother would certainly have taken action, but because her symptoms were so difficult to pin down, and because she herself was incapable of articulating what she was feeling, Nora lost a significant portion of her defining adolescent years to her undiagnosed depression. Now she wanted to be certain that if her depression returned during her pregnancy, she would be able to recognize its symptoms so that she could start treatment as soon as possible.

Had Nora's depression been left untreated much longer, the disease could have robbed her of even more of her life, as it did another patient of mine. Rhoda first began to experience symptoms of depression when she was nineteen years old, and from that point until the age of thirty-four she suffered a depressive episode approximately every two years. Because these episodes seemed to occur mainly during the winter, she was initially diagnosed with seasonal affective disorder (SAD) and told to get away on vacation to warm and sunny places. That worked for a while, but about five years before I met her, the sun was no longer sufficient to elevate her mood, and she began to require a combination of medications just to be functional and feel alive.

In fact, her initial diagnosis is not surprising, since women appear to be three times—with some studies indicating that it's more like four to six times—more vulnerable than men to this relatively common seasonal pattern of depression. While we still do not completely understand the cause, it appears to relate to a dysfunction of the serotonin system, and women with SAD generally suffer intense drowsiness in the daytime despite sleeping long hours at night. They also have carbohydrate cravings, particularly in the afternoon (a phenomenon that has otherwise been associated with a need for the calming effects of serotonin), and tend to gain weight. These seasonal episodes may continue throughout a woman's life, or, as in Rhoda's case, they may develop into a continuous depression.

Survival, for Rhoda, became a daily challenge, and although she wasn't suicidal when she came to see me, she did lament the degree to which her illness had compromised the quality of her life, and she was saddened that an entire decade had been stolen from her, never to be regained.

There's certainly no one cause and no one easy answer to explain why women are statistically at so much greater risk than men or why they seem to manifest symptoms at particular times in their lives. Several researchers have concentrated their studies on various factors and come up with an assortment of biological, psychological, and social issues, any one or a combination of which may be associated with depressive illness in any particular woman.

Biological Factors

Depression and the Family Tree: How Genes Are Passed On

It's been shown that major depression is one and a half to three times more prevalent among those with one or more first-degree blood relatives who have been diagnosed with the problem, and since more women than men are at risk for the disease, it can be considered—even though we do not know exactly how the genetic transmission takes place—that this is one of the less fortunate things daughters may be likely to inherit from their mothers, fathers, or sometimes even grandparents.

Rita and Dan were neighbors whose parents were also friends, and they had known each other since high school, so it was no surprise to either of their families when they announced their plans to marry. After the wedding, however, Rita began to grow more and more upset about the amount of money they'd spent, even though both she and Dan had been saving for their big day, and their parents had also been extremely generous about helping them cover expenses. At first Dan was supportive and assured his bride that her concerns were unfounded, but he could see, after six months had passed, that Rita's unrealistic preoccupation with their finances was escalating to the point of obsession.

It was at that point that her mother shared with Dan's mother the information that she herself had been taking antidepressant medication for twenty-five years, that one of her sisters had recently been hospitalized and received electroshock treatment, and that Rita's grandmother had been institutionalized for many years. In all, as it turned out, Rita had more than six family members currently being treated for psychiatric illness. Her mother went on to say that because of the high incidence of emotional illness in the family, she'd been concerned about Rita from the time she was a child and had actually considered it a "bonus" that her daughter's illness didn't manifest itself sooner.

In my own practice, women with a family history of depression or other psychiatric illness often ask whether they should risk having a baby at all because they are concerned both with the possibility of relapse and with their chances of passing the "bad gene" on to their child.

My answer to these worried women is always that even a genetic predisposition does not mean their child will necessarily become a victim of depression; further, emotional illness, in and of itself, should not prevent any woman from having children so long as her doctor is aware of her history and thus prepared to treat her if necessary.

Not knowing about that family history is what can lead to a problem, as it did when I was called in to see a patient at British Columbia Women's Hospital who had given birth three days before and was, according to the nurses, displaying symptoms of elevated mood, hyperactivity, and speediness, racing from room to room and feeling extraordinarily happy. Because there was no indication on her chart of any prenatal consultation, and no partner in the picture to ask, no one at the hospital knew anything about this woman's history. It wasn't until the patient had recovered sufficiently that she was able to convey to the hospital's social worker who'd been assigned to her case that three of her four siblings had a history of bipolar disorder. The pity is that if we'd known, we would have been able to monitor her properly and could have spared her the embarrassment of having a full-blown manic episode in the maternity hospital.

There are many illnesses, including hypertension, cardiovascular disease, and high cholesterol, among others, that have a strong genetic component. When someone sees a new doctor for the first time or checks into a hospital, he or she generally fills out a form that includes this kind of family information as well as his or her own prior medical history. When I started the Reproductive Mental Health Program at my hospital in 1983, I worked for many years to include information about psychiatric illness on the form our patients filled out. The reason, obviously, is not to stigmatize the patient but to alert us to the possibility of the problem manifesting itself during or following her pregnancy, when she may be particularly vulnerable as a result of hormonal changes and emotional stress.

The Hormonal Connection

As we'll be discussing further in the chapter that follows, the rapid shifts in levels of the female reproductive hormones estrogen and progesterone that occur at puberty, premenstrually, during pregnancy, postpartum, and again during perimenopause and menopause have been shown to be associated with changes in mood and, in extreme cases, psychosis. Although the exact mechanism for these changes isn't known, it appears that fluctuations in the woman's hormonal levels affect a variety of neurotransmitter systems in the brain, making her particularly vulnerable to psychological and emotional problems, specifically depression, at these particular times.

DEPRESSION IN PUBERTY: THE THIEF OF YOUNG GIRLS' LIVES

Various studies have shown that many women experience the onset of depression at the time of adolescence, some as young as ten years of age, while men, in general, do not become symptomatic until their twenties. At puberty, the female-to-male ratio for depression is two to one. This is a time when many girls are struggling with issues of self-image, a time when the development of secondary sexual characteristics can lead to competitiveness, rivalry among peers, and a complex range of emotions that make it difficult for some adolescent girls to cope with the stresses of their lives.

In recent years there have been several groundbreaking books written about what happens to girls psychologically and emotionally as they reach adolescence. Professor Carol Gilligan's *In a Different Voice* discusses the differences between the ways girls and boys develop their sense of identity; Peggy Orenstein's *Schoolgirls* talks about the precipitous drop in self-esteem experienced by so many adolescent girls; *Reviving Ophelia,* by clinical psychologist Mary Pipher, recounts the serious psychological and emotional stumbling blocks encountered by her adolescent patients; and, most recently, Rachel Simmons investigates the insidious, soul-crushing ways in which teenage girls can be mean to one another in *Odd Girl Out.* It should be noted that all of this emotional turmoil is occurring just at the time when girls are experiencing hormonal shifts that also radically affect their mood states.

Girls who develop sexually earlier than their peers may be at in-creased risk for adolescent-onset depression, and it has been found that adolescent girls who have poor parental attachment tend to be more anxious and fail to develop reasonable coping skills, which can then lead to problems with future attachments and eventually to depression.

While it is difficult to untangle the complex interplay of cause and effect between physical and psychological factors, or to equate one de-velopmental stage to another, it would seem reasonable to postulate that the hormonal changes, as well as issues related to body image and the stresses on intimate relationships that occur during puberty, can cre-ate or exacerbate the circumstances that seem to put adolescent girls so at risk for depression.

PREMENSTRUAL DYSPHORIC DISORDER (PMDD)

Premenstrual dysphoric disorder (PMDD) is a severe form of PMS that affects between 3 and 8 percent of women, beginning in their early twenties and peaking in their thirties. Its symptoms typically appear af-ter ovulation, when there is a shift in the ratio of estrogen to proges-terone levels, and continue until the onset of menstruation (or, in some women, through the first three days of the menstrual period). Although first described as "premenstrual tension" by New York gynecologist Dr. Robert T. Frank in 1931, it was not until 1994 that a more specific defi-nition of PMDD was included in the appendix of the *Diagnostic and Statistical Manual of Mental Disorders.*

DSM-IV-TR DIAGNOSTIC CRITERIA FOR
PREMENSTRUAL DYSPHORIC DISORDER

A. In most menstrual cycles during the past year, five of the
   following symptoms are present for most of the time during the
   last week of the luteal phase (before menses), and are entirely
   absent for at least one week postmenses.

   1. Depressed mood, feelings of hopelessness, or self-
      deprecating thoughts

2. Anxiety and tension
3. Affective lability (feeling suddenly sad or tearful or increased sensitivity to rejection)
4. Anger or irritability or increased interpersonal conflicts
5. Decreased interest in usual activities
6. Difficulty concentrating
7. Lethargy, easy fatigability
8. Change in appetite, overeating, or food cravings
9. Hypersomnia or insomnia
10. Sense of being overwhelmed or out of control
11. Breast tenderness, swelling, bloating, weight gain

B. The disturbance markedly interferes with work or school or other activities and relationships.

Adapted from the American Psychiatric Association, *Diagnostic and Statistical Manual of Mental Disorders*, 4th ed., Text Revision (DSM-IV-TR) (Washington, D.C.: American Psychiatric Association, 2000).

For a woman to be diagnosed with PMDD she must exhibit at least five of the above symptoms, including at least one core symptom, for at least one week before menstruation in two consecutive months, and the symptoms must be resolved within a few days of or when her period begins.

In a recent survey of more than one thousand menstruating women between the ages of eighteen and forty-nine, more than half of those who worked reported that their ability to do their job was affected premenstrually, and a significant portion of them reported that their symptoms were severe enough to cause them to miss at least one day of work.

When I started my practice almost no one took PMDD seriously, but since that time there has been much more research into this truly debilitating condition not only at our own PMS clinic under the direction of Dr. Diana Carter but also on an international scale in the United States and in Europe. It now seems clear that, although it is cyclical in nature, PMDD can adversely affect all aspects of a woman's life in much the same way as depression; moreover, it has been shown that after experiencing repeated episodes, those who are predisposed will eventually develop a major depressive disorder.

It has been theorized—and substantiated by the results of at least one study—that the brains of these women are responding abnormally to normal hormonal fluctuations. When study subjects were injected with a synthetic gonadotropin-releasing hormone (GnRH) (which, in effect, works to shut off the chemical changes that occur in the brain as a result of hormonal changes), their symptoms were significantly decreased.

Hormone treatment with both oral contraceptives and progesterone was tried in the 1980s but found to be largely ineffective. More recently, however, various antidepressants, including Prozac (fluoxetine), Paxil (paroxetine), Zoloft (sertraline), Celexa (citalopram), and Effexor (venlafaxine), are proving to be helpful in the treatment of PMDD.

Lola, a thirty-one-year-old mother of two, was referred to the PMS clinic at Women's Hospital for assessment of her hormonally related mood swings because, ever since the birth of her first child four years before, she'd noticed that from the fourteenth to the twenty-eighth day of her menstrual cycle she was extremely angry and irritable, would scream at her children for no reason, and was regularly having to call her husband to leave work and come home to deal with the crisis. In her case, the term "raging hormones" would not have been an exaggeration!

After charting her symptoms through two cycles, it was apparent that Lola really was extremely dysfunctional for fourteen days out of every month. She was prescribed 12.5 mg of Paxil CR to be taken just during that period (from ovulation to menstruation). Her symptoms of PMDD disappeared.

DEPRESSION ASSOCIATED WITH PERIMENOPAUSE AND MENOPAUSE

Menopause is defined by the complete cessation of menstrual periods for the period of one year, while perimenopause is the period of transition prior to menopause when women, typically between the ages of forty-five and fifty, are still menstruating but are experiencing irregularities in their menstrual cycle as a result of decreased or fluctuating hormonal function.

One epidemiological study indicates that the risk of depression actually decreases for women after the age of fifty, while another that was
longitudinal in nature showed no association between natural menopause and depression. When it comes to perimenopause, however, the
jury is apparently still out. Some studies show an increased prevalence
of depressive mood, while others do not. What does seem to be true,
however, is that the longer perimenopause lasts, the greater the chance
that the woman will experience depression.

It should be noted that this period of hormonal change is generally
accompanied by other stresses, such as children leaving or returning
home, having to care for elderly parents, and approaching retirement.
While, again, the relationship between these biological and psychosocial factors has not been objectively substantiated, the perimenopausal
years are yet one more period in a woman's life when a confluence of internal and external change appears to put her at increased risk. And it is
also true that women who have a history of PMDD, postpartum depression, or other, nonhormonal depressive episodes appear to be at greater
risk for experiencing perimenopausal or menopausal depressive illness.

Marlene, for example, at age forty-nine, was going through the perimenopausal transition and struggling with depression and anxiety. She
had been my patient fifteen years earlier, when I had treated her for
postpartum depression associated with the birth of her daughter. At that
time she responded successfully to supportive therapy in combination
with antidepressant medication and had remained on the medication
for a period of two years. After that, she had continued to be stable
without medication until she reached perimenopause.

Now she was extremely irritable and experiencing mood swings as
well as hot flashes and decreased sex drive. Marlene told me that her
consumption of vodka had been increasing steadily over the past couple
of years and that she was "fed up" with dealing with her now-teenage
daughter's PMS. She knew that the depression had come back to haunt
her again. I referred her to another doctor at our hospital who special-
izes in addictions and mental health, and she was treated with Prozac, the
same antidepressant medication to which she had responded earlier. With
the medication and counseling she was able to control her excessive

drinking and get relief from depressive symptoms, and that relief, quite naturally, also allowed her to cope more effectively with her daughter's PMS.

Because of the elevated risks for breast cancer, cardiovascular disease, and other diseases found by the Women's Health Initiative study to be associated with hormone replacement therapy, antidepressants remain the treatment of choice for depression in perimenopausal and menopausal women.

Psychosocial Factors

Even in the United States, it is not unusual for many women to believe that they have no right to express their emotions and that they simply need to "grin and bear it" no matter how bad they may feel. Men, on the other hand, are socialized from an early age to be assertive and aggressive. Not only does this allow them to ask for what they need or want, but it also permits them to find physical outlets generally unavailable to women for resolving their feelings rather than allowing them to fester and deepen. The more isolated and alone the woman feels, the less likely she will be to ask for help, making her risk for depression that much greater.

Crying Out in Silence: Cultural Isolation

Kim is a shy young Korean mother who recently immigrated to North America with her husband and extended family. For a year or more, as her sadness grew and her mood deteriorated, she struggled unsuccessfully to acclimate to her new country. Although she'd tried to talk to her husband about her feelings, he brushed them aside as a "phase" that would pass as she became better adjusted. After that, ashamed and embarrassed that she couldn't be happy in her new home, and assuming—perhaps hoping against hope—that her sad feelings would just go away, she simply lapsed into silence. It wasn't until a neighbor, who one day saw her walking with her baby very close to the riverbank in her town, became alarmed by what seemed to her highly unusual behavior and intervened with Kim's husband that she was finally able to get the help she needed.

While Kim's situation was certainly exacerbated by her lack of community and inability to speak the language of her adopted country, her reaction was not so very different, as I've said, from that of many women who feel they are "stuck" and don't know how to voice their feelings effectively. And when fear enters the equation, as it does in the presence of physical, sexual, or emotional abuse, it may become even harder to seek help.

Victims of Violence

For women who are victims of violence, feelings of guilt and/or helplessness are almost always entwined with feelings of sadness, and their depression, therefore, becomes that much more confusing and difficult for them to recognize or voice.

Nina is a slim, beautiful blonde who, at the age of twenty-one, was naively seduced into marrying a wealthy and powerful man twenty years her senior. As his third wife, Nina was to her husband just one more "acquisition." He took pleasure in showing her off to his friends and colleagues, but in private he belittled her, abused her emotionally, insulted her, and in general made sure she understood that for him she was nothing more than an object. Mercifully, he soon tired of his newest "trophy" and consequently discarded her, but it took Nina several years to regain her sense of self-worth and recover from the depression of believing that she deserved whatever punishment she had received.

Although she surely didn't realize it at the time, Nina was lucky that her destructive marriage didn't last, because when a woman is involved in an abusive relationship and can see no way out, the cycle of abuse and depression becomes truly vicious. In fact, many studies have shown that recovery from depression takes longer when a woman is (or believes herself to be) trapped in a bad relationship.

Elsie was thirty years old, ten weeks pregnant, and bruised both mentally and physically when she arrived in the emergency room of the hospital where I work. Her husband, Rodney, was a bouncer at a local club who apparently enjoyed practicing his profession on his wife. She'd made several attempts to leave the relationship but—like many women in her situation—kept on returning to Rodney until one night, in an uncontrollable rage, he beat her up badly, shouted obscenities, and told her to leave. That's when she finally called 911 and was taken to the hospital, where I happened to be on call.

Even today, I have a vivid recollection of Elsie's sad story of depression made worse by physical abuse and the unimaginable humiliation she suffered at the hands of another human being. The vicious cycle of depression, abuse, and depression continued as Rodney, despite counseling for anger management, was unable to change his behavior. In the end, it was only with intensive therapy that Elsie was finally able to gather the courage to leave with her then-newborn baby once and for all. But the scars, both mental and physical, were, as she told me, very difficult to heal.

Even if a woman's spouse is not overtly abusive or directly responsible for his wife's depression, he may—like Kim's husband—be unwilling or unable to give her the support she needs to get well. To complicate matters even further, women who are currently in supportive and perfectly happy relationships but who were the victims of childhood sexual abuse may be depressed without recognizing the source of their suffering because they have repressed or "forgotten" what happened to them until their memory suddenly returns at a particular moment in their lives, which may well be when they become pregnant or after the baby is born. Childhood sexual abuse is, in fact, a powerful stressor that is known to put women like my patient Daisy at risk for depression later in life.

I met Daisy when she was forty years old and was referred to my office for the treatment of infertility-related depression. She told me that she hadn't thought about the childhood abuse she'd experienced for many years until one day her father came to visit her and she had a sudden flashback. In her mind's eye, she saw her bedroom door opening slowly and her father entering her room, trying to lie down next to her in bed, and touching her inappropriately. As she then went on to explain to me, his abusive behavior had continued for many years until, at the age of seventeen, she finally put a lock on her door and threatened to report him to the police.

One may wonder how anyone could "forget" such an experience, but the human brain has truly amazing capabilities and often tries to protect us from thoughts or feelings that may be too difficult for us to handle. In Daisy's case, it was her infertility treatment, which involved repeated pelvic examinations along with fluctuating hormone levels, that finally triggered her long-repressed memory of childhood sexual abuse.

The Stresses of Single and Working Mothers

If a bad or abusive relationship, past or present, is known to put women at risk for depression, there is also substantial evidence to indicate that motherhood, even for women in what would be considered normal relationships, can be stressful. This is particularly true for working women, who will have to return to work in order to contribute to the family's support but will also, at the same time, be taking care of their child's needs as well as their husband's, putting food on the table, and cleaning the house—most often with little or no assistance from "the man of the family."

Those same stresses are even greater for single mothers. There is evidence to show that single mothers—whether they are separated, divorced, or never married—are three times more likely than married mothers to experience a depressive episode. If a woman is the sole support of her family, working long hours (at a salary that is likely to be less than a male counterpart would receive for doing the same job), then coming home to care for her children, with no opportunity to socialize or communicate with others, is it any wonder that the ongoing unrelieved stress would eventually lead to depression?

But there's more. For reasons that are not entirely clear, single women are also more likely to be those who have experienced childhood adversities related to socioeconomic deprivation, which increase their risk for depression. Once again, cause and effect appear to travel in a vicious cycle: when experiences in childhood militate against women's ability to develop fulfilling adult relationships, women are put at greater risk for depression, a risk that is in turn further increased by their being on their own in a stressful life situation.

The Depression of Bereavement

One of the greatest stressors we can experience in life is the loss of a loved one, be it a parent, a spouse, or a child. The loss of a child is, of course, a cruel and devastating event for anyone, male or female, and fraught with complicated bereavement issues, but for the simple reason that women are statistically more likely to live longer, they are also more likely than men to be suffering the stress associated with the loss of a spouse. And studies show that in general they also take longer than men to recover from a trauma of this nature.

Furthermore, when the death is sudden, as it was for Darlene's husband, the trauma is compounded, and so is the likelihood that it will trigger a depressive episode, or the recurrence of a previous depression.

Both Darlene and her husband were fifty-four years old when tragedy struck. They were driving home together one evening and had stopped at an intersection when Darlene looked over at her husband in the driver's seat and saw that he was holding on to the wheel with his eyes shut tight. Assuming that he'd fallen asleep at the wheel, she was concerned but not too alarmed as she reached over to wake him up. The horror set in when she realized he wasn't breathing; he'd died instantly of a sudden heart attack. In that moment Darlene's life changed forever, and the trauma, understandably, sent her into an emotional tailspin.

Although Darlene appeared to be biologically predisposed to depression and had previously been treated for that illness, she'd been doing well without any medication for several years. Now, however, she was plunged back into that dark place where, as she described it, she felt like "a victim chained to feelings of sadness." In this instance, Darlene's depression was clearly triggered by the stress of her bereavement, but not everyone who experiences the loss of a spouse is destined to become depressed, and in her case, the relapse was undoubtedly compounded by her biological predisposition. It's important to remember that in most

instances there is a constellation of reasons or causes even for circum-
stantial depression.

More Common but Also More Complex: The Gender Gap

Not only do psychosocial and biological factors put women at greater
risk than men for depression, but the women who suffer this disease
seem to do so differently and in conjunction with more secondary conditions that can make them more difficult to treat.

Many studies indicate that at least some women seem to demonstrate what is defined by the DSM-IV-TR as atypical depression, which is
characterized by increased drowsiness, increased appetite, rejection sensitivity, and, finally, leaden paralysis. In addition, they tend to have
more cravings for chocolate and other carbohydrates, and seem to gain
weight, whereas men, in general, do not have food cravings but rather experience loss of appetite, lose weight, and report a lack of sleep.
Women also recover more slowly and experience more recurrences of
the disease than do men.

Perhaps because their symptoms are different, men and women respond differently to a variety of antidepressant medications. Men, for
example, respond better than women to tricyclic antidepressants, while
women do better on monoamine oxidase inhibitors (MAOIs) and selective serotonin reuptake inhibitors (SSRIs). One explanation for both the
differences in symptoms and the differences in response to medication
would seem to be the role played by hormonal changes in women's depressive illness. Studies have shown that while perimenopausal women respond better to the SSRI Zoloft (sertraline) than do men, postmenopausal
women do better (and as well as men) on Tofranil (imipramine), which
is a tricyclic antidepressant—probably because the hormonal status of
postmenopausal women is similar to that of men. And both peri- and
postmenopausal women on hormone replacement therapy (HRT) appear to do better on Prozac (fluoxetine) than those who are not.

Women's treatment, moreover, is often complicated by the fact that
more women than men suffer other conditions that accompany and

complicate their depression. Fifty-one percent, for example, suffer some form of anxiety disorder—including panic disorder, generalized anxiety disorder, and obsessive-compulsive disorder—in conjunction with major depression. But it is not only adjunctive psychological disorders that make women more difficult to treat. They are also more likely than men to suffer from medical conditions such as arthritis and migraine headaches, and the combination of migraine and depression in particular is a major challenge to treat. Since migraines are often related to hormonal changes. I personally have treated many patients for whom migraines and depression form a lethal combination. Sheila was one of those patients.

When Sheila failed to keep her appointment for the third time, I called her at home. Her husband answered the phone and explained in a whisper that for the past four days his wife had been lying in a quiet dark room, curtains drawn, suffering a horrible migraine. She had already been taking 25 mg of Paxil CR, one of the newer selective serotonin reuptake inhibitors, and had initially had some relief from her symptoms. But for the past three months, following the birth of her child six months before, her severe premenstrual migraines had returned. Her treatment plan included seeing a neurologist, increasing her Paxil CR to 40 mg premenstrually, and strict adherence to diet. (In addition to hormones, foods and altitude changes can also trigger migraine headaches.)

Depression in Women: A Confluence of Causes

With all the evidence at our disposal, it seems clear that more than coincidence is involved when women experience depressive mood disorders at critical times of change in their reproductive biology. These normal biological changes, beginning with puberty in their early teens and continuing through menopause in their fifties, put women at risk for recurrent depression through most of their adult lives. What is more, the biological changes associated with depression in women are also associated with times of particular stress in their lives. What all of these factors should tell us is not only that treating women requires us to be sensitive to both the physical and emotional changes they are experiencing but also that pregnancy, a time of mental and emotional stress as well as major biological change, is a turning point when women will be particularly vulnerable to depression.

In the following chapter we'll look more closely at exactly how hormones as well as the neurotransmitters that affect mood are released in the brain and how changes in one appear to affect and create changes in the other.

3

Neurotransmitters, Hormones, and Depression

Today, we hear a lot about the fact that depression is caused by a chemical imbalance. Those chemicals are neurotransmitters, "messengers" released in specific areas of the brain that cause us to react mentally, emotionally, and physically to what's going on in our internal and external environment. The "imbalance" refers to the variations in their concentration that appear to play a significant role in a variety of mental disorders including not only depression but also schizophrenia, Parkinson's disease, and others. Although there are certainly a number of factors that determine why one person becomes depressed while another does not, the one thing we know that all depressed people have in common is altered levels of neurotransmitters.

Therefore, to further understand how genetics and biology may interface with psychosocial stress factors to trigger depression in women, we need to take a look inside the brain.

A Look Inside the Brain

Clearly, the structure and function of the human brain are not subjects to be explained in one short chapter, nor is doing that the purpose of this book. That said, however, any real understanding of why some women are at an increased risk for becoming depressed at particular junctures in their lives requires some basic knowledge of how the brain works.

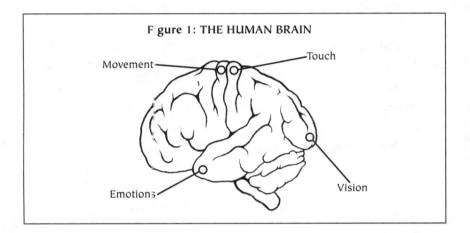

Figure 1: THE HUMAN BRAIN

Movement

Touch

Emotions

Vision

Our human brain contains more than ten billion cells, called neurons or nerve cells, that "talk" to one another by sending signals back and forth via brain chemicals called neurotransmitters. By doing that (in the course of conversation, so to speak), these nerve cells determine all of our voluntary and involuntary actions and reactions. If one cell needs to communicate information to another, it releases neurotransmitters

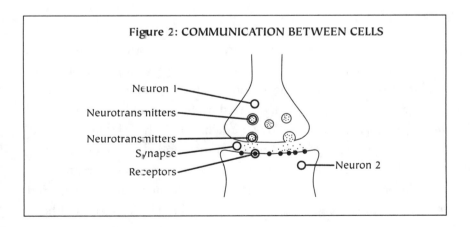

Figure 2: COMMUNICATION BETWEEN CELLS

Neuron 1

Neurotransmitters

Neurotransmitters

Synapse

Receptors

Neuron 2

into the space between the cells, called the synapse. The neurotransmitters then deliver messages to the adjoining cell by attaching themselves to the cell's receptors. Each neurotransmitter has its own particular receptor, and together the two work like a key fitting into a lock. If the key doesn't fit, the lock won't turn. In terms of the brain, this means that signals won't get crossed, and messages will get delivered to the right place.

We have more than a hundred neurotransmitters in our brain, but the four that have been shown to be associated with depression (and, therefore, the ones we'll be talking about here) are serotonin, norepinephrine, dopamine, and acetylcholine. Gamma-aminobutyric acid (GABA) has also recently been receiving attention and appears to be implicated in the occurrence of major depression and PMDD.

Neurotransmitters and Depression

When you are depressed, for reasons science has yet to determine, the availability of one or more of these neurotransmitters is decreased. As a result, the communication between brain cells is impaired. When the amount of available neurotransmitter is returned to normal levels, either naturally or with antidepressant medications, the symptoms of depression are controlled.

Serotonin

Serotonin is one of the most important neurotransmitters associated with depression, particularly in women, and has an interesting story behind it. It originates from the amino acid tryptophan (a building block of proteins), which was first discovered in the seed pods of the *Griffonia simplicifolia* plant in western Africa. You may have heard that one of the reasons people seem to become so sluggish and sleepy after Thanksgiving dinner is that turkey contains significant amounts of tryptophan. In addition to turkey, however, it is found in many other plant and animal proteins, such as peanuts, soybeans, brown rice, fish, and beef;

humans cannot produce this amino acid themselves and so must get it from food sources. Although tryptophan supplements in pill form are available in Canada, the Food and Drug Administration does not approve them for sale in the United States.

Through complex chemical pathways, our bodies convert tryptophan into serotonin, which has been found to play a critical role in ensuring emotional calmness, restful sleep, the regulation and perception of pain, sexual behavior, and appetite control. In fact, our general level of satisfaction and happiness with the world around us depends largely on our levels of serotonin.

A particular class of antidepressants known as SSRIs, or selective serotonin reuptake inhibitors, which include Prozac (fluoxetine), Paxil (paroxetine), Zoloft (sertraline), Celexa (citalopram), and Lexapro and Cipralex (escitalopram), works by inhibiting the reabsorption of serotonin in the brain cells, thus ensuring that plenty of this particular neurotransmitter is available to regulate your mood.

Norepinephrine

Norepinephrine (noradrenaline) is a neurotransmitter as well as a hormone that controls the stress response or "flight-or-fight" reaction, as it is commonly known. So, for example, when you are frightened and your heart beats fast and you breathe more heavily, this is because your system is pumping large amounts of norepinephrine into your body.

In the 1960s, Dr. Joseph Schildkraut of Harvard University was the first to make the connection between mood and neurotransmitters. He theorized—as turned out to be true—that depression, or "low mood," was caused by a deficiency of norepinephrine in the brain and, conversely, that an excess of the same neurotransmitter was responsible for mania, or elevated mood.

Among the older classes of antidepressants, those called tricyclics and MAOIs (monoamine oxidase inhibitors) work by increasing the amount of norepinephrine available in the central nervous system (the brain and the spinal cord).

In addition, there is yet another new class of drugs called dual-action antidepressants, which includes Effexor (venlafonaxine) and Remeron (mirtazapine), that work on both norepinephrine and serotonin, thus raising the levels of both these neurotransmitters in the brain.

Dopamine, Acetylcholine, and GABA

Dopamine, the neurotransmitter most commonly associated with the "pleasure system" in the brain, is released to increase levels of pleasure in response to naturally rewarding experiences such as food and sex. This increase in the level of pleasure is exactly what people who get high on cocaine or other dopamine-stimulating drugs are seeking.

In terms of psychiatric illness, too much dopamine is most closely associated with schizophrenia, while a lack of it has been linked to atypical depressions such as seasonal affective disorder and to the depressive symptoms associated with Parkinson's disease. Most researchers believe that whatever role it may play in the onset of depression, dopamine ought to be studied within the context of what we already know about norepinephrine and serotonin.

Like dopamine, acetylcholine is a neurotransmitter that has been suggested to have some responsibility for the onset of depression, but precisely what role it might play still remains unclear at this point. We do know that acetylcholine facilitates good digestion, deeper breathing, and a slower heart rate, all of which are associated with relaxation.

Finally, GABA is an interesting neurotransmitter often referred to as the body's "natural tranquilizer," as it has relaxing properties and a calming effect. Its deficiency causes irritability and insomnia and is linked to depression. Dr. Gerard Sanacora and a team of researchers at Yale University, using brain-imaging techniques, found that GABA levels were significantly reduced in patients with depressive illness.

With relation specifically to women, those who suffer severe premenstrual symptoms also show low levels of GABA in the second half (luteal phase) of their menstrual cycle. And in women with postpartum blues, low GABA seems to be related to low levels of mood.

All of these neurotransmitters are associated with depression in both men and women. In women, however, altered hormone levels also appear to play a role. The female reproductive hormones related to menstruation, conception, and gestation are therefore particularly significant in any discussion of depression in women of childbearing age.

What Are Hormones?

I'm sure everyone at least *thinks* she knows what hormones are. We've all heard the jokes about women "being hormonal," and almost every woman has at some time or another blamed her bad mood or short temper on being premenstrual. But how many women really understand how these hormones work in the body?

Hormones, in fact, work much like neurotransmitters in that they attach to various cells and cause particular effects. Like neurotransmitters, hormones are chemical substances that are critical to regulating a variety of bodily functions, and, as with neurotransmitters, too much or too little of any particular hormone can cause an imbalance that prevents the body from functioning exactly as it should.

As we discussed in the previous chapter, the onset or recurrence of depression in women has been associated with those particular times when hormone levels fluctuate significantly—at puberty, during the various premenstrual phases of the menstrual cycle, during pregnancy, at childbirth, with the onset of perimenopause, and, finally, after menopause.

Your Reproductive Hormones and How They Work

The three main sex hormones (also called steroid hormones), estrogen, progesterone, and testosterone, are all derived from cholesterol through a series of chemical reactions. While estrogen and progesterone are the two that concern us most with regard to mood fluctuations and depression in women, testosterone, to a certain degree, seems to be caught up in the mix as well.

Estrogens

Estrogen is the "feminizing hormone" and affects the various female reproductive organs in critical ways. There are three types of estrogen: 17-beta-estradiol, estrone, and estriol. Estrogens are primarily responsible for:

1. The development of girls into sexually mature women

   - Development of breasts
   - Maturing of the uterus and vagina
   - Broadening of the pelvis
   - Growth of pubic and auxiliary hair
   - Increase and distribution of fat tissue

2. The onset of menstruation and preparation of the body for possible pregnancy
3. The maintenance of pregnancy once conception occurs

The additional effects of estrogen that are not specifically related to reproduction include:

1. Strengthening bones and minimizing loss of calcium
2. Lowering cholesterol levels
3. Preventing hardening of the arteries

Another function of estrogen is to regulate the production of progesterone across the full term of a pregnancy, in addition to which it is vital to the development of the lungs, kidneys, liver, and other important organs in the fetus.

Progesterone

Progesterone is the second female sex hormone that, in conjunction with estrogen, controls menstruation and reproduction. As indicated by the word itself (*pro-*, "in favor of," *-gesterone*, "gestation"), it is the hormone critical to preparing the uterus for and maintaining a pregnancy.

Progesterone causes the lining of the uterus to thicken in preparation for pregnancy. When conception does occur, the structure of the uterine lining changes and the placenta develops. Beginning at the twelfth week of gestation, the placenta starts producing progesterone, which is essential to the maintenance of the pregnancy.

Testosterone

Believe it or not, the female body does produce testosterone—but only a tenth of what men make. Although it is generally (and not entirely accurately) associated with competitive, aggressive males, testosterone is the hormone most responsible for sexual desire in both men and women. The increased sex drive in younger women just prior to ovulation is, in fact, a result of rising testosterone levels, whereas postmenopausal women, who are deficient in this hormone, experience a reduction of their sex drive.

Hormones and Your Menstrual Cycle

Chinese sages referred to the menstrual blood of women as the essence of Mother Earth, the yin principle that gives life to all things. In ancient societies, menstrual blood carried spiritual significance, and while we may no longer imbue it with such supernatural power, we do now understand that the menstrual cycle controls the most complex workings of the female body. During the menstrual cycle, a woman's brain, hormones, and reproductive organs work together in a symphony, with the pituitary gland (located in the brain) acting as the conductor of the orchestra. These perfectly coordinated events occur in most women every twenty-eight days.

From birth, the ovaries contain close to five thousand eggs, each of which is situated in its own sac, or follicle. The hypothalamus—the body's CEO, so to speak—initiates the menstrual cycle by signaling the pituitary to secrete follicle-stimulating hormone (FSH). FSH then stimulates the ovarian follicles to grow and secrete estrogen during the first half of the menstrual cycle and also prepares the uterus to receive the fertilized egg. When estrogen reaches a certain level, it triggers the pituitary to produce lutenizing hormone (LH). When LH levels rise, peaking around the fourteenth day of the twenty-eight-day menstrual cycle, only one follicle (the dominant follicle) matures and releases an egg. This is ovulation.

If the egg is fertilized, the woman becomes pregnant. The fertilized egg attaches to the uterus and begins to grow. Progesterone rises, and you start to feel the early symptoms of pregnancy, such as morning sickness.

However, if the egg is not fertilized, in the second half of the menstrual cycle the corpus luteum (the collapsed follicle) starts to secrete progesterone, which thickens the uterine lining. It is this lining that is eventually shed as your period. Estrogen and progesterone levels then drop, triggering the hypothalamus to start the cycle all over again. This chain of events repeats itself every month.

Figure 3: THE BRAIN, HORMONES, AND THE MENSTRUAL CYCLE

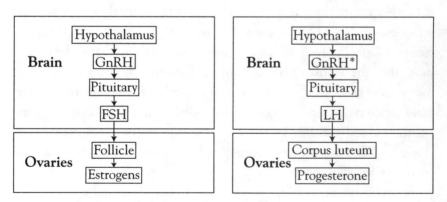

1st Half of Cycle   *2nd Half of Cycle*

*Gonadotropin-releasing hormone

Secondary Reproductive Hormones

Although estrogen and progesterone have the primary responsibility for preparing a woman's body to conceive and bear a child, there are two other reproductive hormones—prolactin and oxytocin—that also play important roles in the process.

Prolactin, the Nursing Hormone

Prolactin causes the secretion of milk from the breast. When conception occurs, prolactin secretion increases, reaching peak levels just prior to birth. About three weeks after delivery, blood levels of prolactin fall to normal. If the woman is breast-feeding, the suckling of the infant again prompts increased prolactin production, but even when a woman is nursing, those levels will naturally decline after about three months.

Prolactin is released from the anterior portion of the pituitary gland, and its production is stimulated in both men and women by an increase in exercise, as well as after surgery or by psychological stress.

Oxytocin, the Birthing Hormone

Oxytocin is the hormone that stimulates uterine contractions during childbirth. It is produced in the hypothalamus and released by the posterior portion of the pituitary gland. If oxytocin secretion begins too soon, it may induce preterm labor and premature birth. When all works as it should, the fetal head pushing through during birth stimulates oxytocin secretion every few minutes in the pulsating rhythm of labor. Then, when the newborn suckles at the nipple, it is again oxytocin that causes ejection of milk for the baby.

In addition to these vital functions, oxytocin is an antianxiety hormone that has a calming effect on the new mother. Not only does this amazing hormone aid in the birthing process, but also it actually enhances the mother's positive feelings toward her baby.

Cortisol and Reproduction

For centuries, physicians have understood that there is a relationship between stress and the reproductive system. As far back as the fifth century BCE, Hippocrates tried to explain the high incidence of impotence among tribes in what is now the Ukraine by relating it to their leading stressful lives. One clear, modern-day example of how stress can affect reproduction is the condition known as amenorrhea, when a woman's menstrual cycle shuts down completely as the result of extreme ongoing anxiety or stress.

A hormone called cortisol, which is secreted by the adrenal glands, situated near the kidneys, regulates this stress response in humans. When we are stressed, small amounts of cortisol secretion are expected and are not harmful to the body. In addition, during the latter half of a pregnancy, there is a natural increase of cortisol in the placenta, which activates the production of progesterone. And, as I've said, it is progesterone that helps to ensure the maintenance of the pregnancy.

With ongoing exposure to stress, however, cortisol is produced continuously, and there is growing evidence that excessive cortisol exposure in pregnancy is in some way responsible for physiological and psychological problems in both the mother and the offspring.

The association between abnormally high levels of cortisol and depression in humans was made in the late 1950s, but it's only in the past ten years that we have understood how it affects women's reproductive functions. As the result of a variety of stressors, both physical and psychological—for example, during pregnancy—normal cortisol levels can increase. In fact, when a woman is unusually anxious or depressed, progesterone itself can be converted into cortisol.

While the connections among cortisol, mood, and pregnancy are unclear, it is important to understand that excessive cortisol in the mother's blood during pregnancy can also reach the fetus through the placenta, with negative effects in the fetus and newborn. (I'll be discussing these effects in detail in Chapter 11.) However, to date researchers have mainly established the relationship between the cortisol "crash" postpartum and the onset of postpartum depression.

The Mothering Brain

The complex interaction of neurotransmitters and hormones creates a cascade of changes in a woman's brain that prepare her for childbirth and motherhood. Estrogen and progesterone act to prepare the womb for conception and maintain the pregnancy, and cortisol aids in the production of progesterone, while oxytocin and prolactin facilitate birthing and nursing.

When this cascade of cause and effect is disturbed at any point, that disruption will have a significant effect on the entire process. In recent years, however, we have begun to understand that there is also a strong link between changes in the levels of hormonal production and disruption of the neurotransmitters that modulate mood during pregnancy and postpartum.

Reproductive Hormones, Neurotransmitters, and Moods

Pregnancy, as we've already discussed, is a time when hormone levels, stress, and mood are likely to have a profound effect on one another. The fact is, however, that all women experience the same increase in estrogen and progesterone levels during pregnancy, but only 10 to 12 percent of these women will suffer from depression in pregnancy. The question that scientists still need to answer, then, is how this 10 to 12 percent may differ biochemically from the majority, whose mood remains stable.

It seems likely that among those who are genetically predisposed, the constant fluctuation in hormone levels throughout the forty weeks of pregnancy may disrupt production of the neurotransmitters that regulate mood. And, as we'll be discussing in the following chapters, external stress factors (including the stress of pregnancy itself) may interact with these women's internal biochemistry to exacerbate the risk for depression.

Low estrogen levels have been associated with depression in women. While the explanation of how this happens is not straightforward, we do know that high estrogen levels increase norepinephrine and sero-tonin activity in the brain, which contributes to positive mood. We also know that a reduction in estrogen levels triggers the brain to release monoamine oxidase (MAO), the enzyme that breaks down and destroys the "feel-good" neurotransmitter serotonin.

In summary, happy mood equals high levels of serotonin and norepi-nephrine. Thus, an acute deficiency of serotonin after the birth of the baby (when estrogen levels fall) could explain, at least in part, why some women experience postpartum depression.

In one study, Dr. Alain Gregoire and colleagues in the United King-dom showed that women who were treated with estrogen patches fol-lowing the onset of a major depression in the early postpartum months responded positively to this treatment. Their findings support the notion that estrogen deficiency could be one of the components contributing to the onset of postpartum depression. And in another study published in the *American Journal of Psychiatry*, Dr. Lee Cohen, Dr. Deborah Sichel, and colleagues gave a one-month course of estrogen beginning immediately after delivery to women who had histories of postpartum mood disorders—some even of postpartum psychosis—and found that most of their subjects did not relapse. So estrogen may also have a pre-ventative effect on a select population of women who are at risk for post-partum depression.

In pregnancy, estrogen levels rise to 130 times their normal levels. With the results of these studies at hand, and knowing what we do about the relationship between estrogen levels and the production of both norepinephrine and serotonin, we might logically assume that these increased levels would protect women from feeling depressed during pregnancy. But in reality, that is not the case.

Does this mean, then, that increased estrogen levels are also related to the onset of depression in some *predisposed* pregnant women? While this does seem to be the case, the precise relationship between increased estrogen and the onset of depression during pregnancy still remains something of a mystery. The answer, however, may lie with the simulta-neous rise in progesterone levels.

Progesterone levels rise sevenfold during pregnancy. In the past,

scientists had thought that progesterone, like estrogen, had antidepressant qualities, but newer research has found that progesterone actually promotes the breakdown of serotonin. Although levels of serotonin in pregnant depressed women have not been measured directly, studies have shown a correlation between depressed mood and high levels of progesterone in pregnancy. For example, Dr. Beverly Pearson Murphy and colleagues at McGill University measured the levels of progesterone metabolites in 203 pregnant women and then screened them for depression. Seven percent of the 203 were found to meet the diagnostic criteria for major depression, and *the same 7 percent* were also found to have higher levels of progesterone metabolites than those who were not depressed, indicating that increased progesterone levels are associated with mood changes during pregnancy.

Dr. J. Galen Buckwalter and colleagues from the University of Southern California also measured levels of progesterone in women during pregnancy and postpartum and found that during pregnancy, high levels of progesterone were associated with increased mood disturbances. In summary, then, although we don't know exactly how this works, increased progesterone levels would seem to be a factor for at least some pregnant depressed women.

In addition to the fluctuations in progesterone and estrogen levels during pregnancy and postpartum, changes in the levels of testosterone during this time are also thought to affect mood. Dr. Buckwalter and his colleagues, in addition to measuring progesterone, also measured levels of testosterone after delivery and found that its increase was strongly and consistently associated with an increase in reported mood disturbances. Yet another study, this one conducted by Dr. Maria Hohlagschwandtner and her colleagues at the University Hospital in Vienna, found that increased levels of testosterone during pregnancy were associated with depressed mood as well as increased irritability and anger. Thus it appears that the male hormone, testosterone, also plays a role in depression among both pregnant and postpartum women.

Despite these findings, for most women the rise and fall of hormone levels in pregnancy and after delivery do not lead to clinical depression. And so, simplistic as this may sound, at present the most likely explanation for why some women become depressed while others do not would seem to be that each woman's brain is wired in a unique way. Just as some of us are hardwired to be shy or gregarious, scientifically inclined or musical, it appears that this same kind of wiring causes a significant minority of women to respond to the interplay of hormones and neurotransmitters in a way that triggers severe mood disturbances.

4

Depression in Pregnancy

THE HORMONE-STRESS CONNECTION

Given what we've already learned about the links among female hormones, neurotransmitters, and stress in terms of the risk for depression, it sometimes amazes me that we're still so resistant to recognizing how widespread and devastating pregnancy-related depression truly is among women today.

Because there have not yet been any studies of large populations, we are relying on research done in clinics, obstetrical hospitals, and highly specialized, hospital-based outpatient centers to provide us with estimates of the frequency with which this debilitating and dangerous condition occurs—and those figures vary widely, from as low as 8 percent to as high as 51 percent. In one paper, reviewing a number of studies related to the prevalence of depression in pregnancy, Heather Bennett and colleagues at the University of Toronto found that on average 7.4 percent of women were reported to suffer from depression during the first trimester of their pregnancy. In the second trimester, that figure rose to 12.8 percent, and in the third trimester, frequency was reported at 12 percent. Yet the *Diagnostic and Statistical Manual of Mental Disorders (DSM-IV-TR)*, the "bible" of all recognized psychiatric illnesses, does not make any reference at all to depression during pregnancy.

Overall, however, I believe we must assume that it is widely unrecognized and therefore dangerously underreported. One reason for this may be the way the illness is diagnosed.

The diagnosis of depression depends largely on the symptoms reported by the patient and the doctor's assessment of those symptoms. Although there are several screening tools available, including self-rating questionnaires for the patient to complete as well as rating systems doctors can use to evaluate their patients' responses to such simple questions as "How is your mood today?" or "How has your mood been in the last week or so?" (for more on this see Appendix), it appears that a substantial proportion of women still go undiagnosed. In fact, a Swedish study of approximately 1,734 pregnant women selected at random determined not only that 14 percent showed symptoms of psychiatric disorders but also that a majority of those had gone undiagnosed and untreated up to that point. While clinicians are vigilant about screening for pregnancy-related medical conditions—as well they should be—they still, by and large, seem to overlook or ignore the state of their patients' emotional well-being.

It appears that too many medical practitioners may continue to be influenced by the traditional belief that pregnancy is somehow "protective" against mood disorders, a belief that stems, no doubt, from two serious misconceptions—that the rise in estrogen levels during pregnancy will keep women "happy" and that impending motherhood is somehow guaranteed to be a wonderfully positive experience.

Compounding this initial bias is the fact that many obstetricians with heavy caseloads spend very little time with their patients. So if depression isn't on their radar screen, so to speak, it won't be high on their list of issues to address during the short time they have with each patient. They will certainly monitor for the fetal heartbeat, take a urine sample, and check for weight gain, but rarely will they ask about the woman's mental health, even though mental health is, without doubt, as important as physical health for both the mother-to-be and the fetus. And, sadly, not many women who *are* depressed will voluntarily share their emotional problems with their doctor. In fact, when they are depressed they may be inclined to avoid prenatal care altogether.

Because depression causes the sufferer to become withdrawn and dis-interested in life, many women who are depressed during pregnancy will fail to schedule or repeatedly cancel visits to their doctor. They may neglect or jeopardize their own health and nutrition, even self-medicate with alcohol or drugs, and by doing so they may also jeopardize the health of their unborn child. Furthermore, antenatal depression is often a precursor or predictor of postpartum depression.

The Pregnancy-Postpartum Continuum

For years we didn't pay very much attention to the connection between antenatal and postpartum depression, but more recently both research-ers and caregivers have started to become aware of the fact that a con-tinuum truly does exist.

In 1982 and again in 1984, two separate studies—the first by J. L. Cox and colleagues and the second by A. K. Atkinson and colleagues—reported that an anxious or depressed mood during pregnancy might presage postpartum depression.

Then, in a groundbreaking study, the results of which were pub-lished as far back as 1989, Dr. Ian Gotlib of Ontario, Canada, assessed more than 350 women for depressive symptoms both during pregnancy and after delivery. The first assessment was done at about twenty-three weeks of gestation, the second at approximately thirty-five weeks, and the last at about four months postpartum. At the first assessment, 21.5 percent of these women were found to be suffering from depressive symptoms. By the second assessment, that number had grown to 25.8 percent, and at the final assessment, 24.8 percent were found to be depressed.

Whether more women became depressed as their pregnancy pro-gressed or whether the symptoms presented by some were not pro-nounced enough to become obvious until the second assessment is not entirely clear. What is clear, however, is that if depression goes un-treated during pregnancy, it will worsen and more than likely continue postpartum. In fact, Dr. Gotlib reported that more than 50 percent of his patients diagnosed in the postpartum period had actually experienced the onset of depression during pregnancy. Unfortunately, we too often recognize this pregnancy-related onset only in retrospect.

When Deena, a young mother of two, was pregnant with her third child, her depression was so severe that her symptoms were obvious and easily diagnosed even by my student who hadn't yet completed his training in medicine, much less psychiatry. Sadly, however, her illness by that time was so firmly entrenched that she required hospitalization. It was only during her hospital stay, when we were able to speak with her over a period of time, that we came to realize she'd actually had less serious depressions during and following both of her previous pregnancies. The question then became, why hadn't someone recognized Deena's depression sooner and possibly prevented her from suffering so long?

Unfortunately, because her family had disapproved of her pregnancies—believing that she was "too young" and needed to complete her education before she started having babies—they'd effectively cut her out of their lives, which meant that she had very little contact with anyone except her partner, Larry, who, while well-meaning and supportive, was also very young and naive about what Deena was going through. As a result, there was really no one there to step in and see that she got the help she needed before she became sick enough to require hospitalization.

I can certainly understand that because I too, early in my career, when I was much less aware of the prevalence of antenatal depression, missed a diagnosis in one of my own patients until after she had given birth. Rowena had been admitted to the hospital because of serious medical complications during her pregnancy, and when her mood began to decline dramatically, I was called in to see her. But despite the fact that I had ample opportunity to speak with her one-on-one for long periods of time, I didn't see what was right before my eyes.

After she'd given birth and was medically stabilized, Rowena attempted suicide. Only then, treating her and looking back at her history, did I realize she'd been depressed throughout her pregnancy. In fact, she told me then that she herself had been aware of her illness but had been too ashamed and embarrassed to "bother" her doctors with her emotional complaints at a time when her medical situation was so serious.

The point here is that we health care providers need to be more vigilant about recognizing depressive symptoms during pregnancy so that we can manage the illness and perhaps prevent it from continuing in the postnatal period.

In one particular study designed to confirm the link between antenatal and postpartum depression, Dr. Jonathon Evans and his colleagues in the Division of Psychiatry at the University of Bristol, England, used a screening tool called the Edinburgh Postnatal Depression Scale (see Appendix, page 253) to examine 9,028 women at four different times: at eighteen and thirty-two weeks of pregnancy and again at eight weeks and eight months postpartum. Significantly, 14 percent were shown to have probable depression at thirty-two weeks of pregnancy as compared to only 9.1 percent at eight weeks postpartum. In addition, the researchers determined that the self-reported depressive symptoms were higher during pregnancy than postpartum; moreover, the severity and nature of the depression were the same before and after childbirth.

The question then remains whether there is a cultural, ethnic, or socioeconomic link that would put some women more at risk than others. The answer to that is both yes and no. There are certainly collateral problems that would increase a woman's probability for depression, and the illness is better recognized and, therefore, more frequently diagnosed in some cultures than in others, but that doesn't mean it can't (or doesn't) affect women of all cultures, in all socioeconomic groups, and at all educational levels. In fact, ironically, when a woman's life has been going well and her expectations for perfection are high, her need to continue being "perfect" during pregnancy, as well as her unrealistically exaggerated fear that "something may go wrong," can sometimes actually trigger stress-related depression.

An Illness Without Borders

Each year I return to my native India to help educate my medical colleagues there about the need for assessing patients for depression. But it hasn't been easy. Many of them simply cannot understand why any woman who had planned a pregnancy and was looking forward to giving birth could possibly be depressed. "What is depression, after all?" they ask. "Sometimes you feel unhappy, and feeling unhappy is normal. Why are you making such a big deal out of it?"

Does this mean there are fewer women in India suffering from antenatal depression than there are in other parts of the world? Frankly, I doubt it. To me it means simply that in India, as in other developing countries throughout the world, thousands of women may simply ignore the illness, as do their health care providers. When I spoke about antenatal depression at the annual psychiatric meeting in India recently, I could see that my audience needed plenty of convincing about the frequency and seriousness of a problem that is now becoming a leading public health concern in the United States. What I also realized, however, is that in some developing countries, such as India and many African nations, poverty is a much larger issue than depression. In this century, this is a pity!

One study of six hundred women in Taiwan found that 8.7 percent had experienced depression during pregnancy and 14 percent suffered postpartum depression, numbers similar to those we have found in North America. Unfortunately, however, very few such geographically specific studies have been done, particularly in countries that are still developing and economically disadvantaged. And while I am certainly in a position to be more aware than most of how different the concerns of these countries are from our own, I am also, as a psychiatrist, exquisitely aware of the degree to which untold numbers of women are suffering without any recognition or relief from their pain.

One area in which we are making some progress, however, is in the study of minority and immigrant populations in North America.

Depression Among Minority and Immigrant Populations

Among minority groups, one study of African American and Hispanic women living in urban poverty completed by social workers at the Albert Einstein College of Medicine in New York showed that depression peaked in the third trimester of pregnancy among those who had poor social support. Interestingly, the same study also indicated that their method of coping with any type of conflict tended toward avoidance rather than seeking resolution. While these women's coping style may not be related specifically to their depression, one might extrapolate that their avoidance had prevented them from seeking treatment for their illness.

The U.S. Census for 2000 reports that there are approximately thirty-two million Latinos living in the United States, of whom 66 percent are of Mexican descent. The same census also reported that Latinos of Mexican descent have the highest fertility rate of all racial and ethnic groups in the country. They are often economically disadvantaged and poorly educated; these same women are also often exposed to physical violence and substance abuse and are often less likely to receive proper care. In a study done of three hundred women of Mexican descent (fifty-nine of them pregnant and seventy within six months postpartum) in an urban northern California setting, 51 percent were found to be at risk for depression. Perhaps even more interesting, however, this study and others have also shown a positive correlation between the women's degree of acculturation and their risk for pregnancy-related depression. In another finding, the more acculturated they were, the greater was their risk of giving birth to an underweight baby. In addition, those who were born in the United States and spoke English were more likely to gain excessive weight during pregnancy, to have sexually transmitted diseases, to smoke, to drink alcohol, and to have more prenatal complications than those who were born in Mexico and spoke Spanish.

It might seem counterintuitive that the greater the degree to which a woman has assimilated into her new culture, the greater would be her risk for depression. This research, however, showed that the positive

correlation between acculturation and psychological distress was related to the alienation and discrimination these women experienced in
a society that values individualism and self-reliance—values that stand
in stark contrast to the emphasis placed on family and community in
the Mexican culture.

Yet another study of African American and Hispanic women has
shown that more than a third of those who were experiencing depression during pregnancy had lost someone important to them during the
previous year, had fewer social supports overall, and had experienced
more negative life events than those who were not depressed. Perhaps
even more sadly, it has also been shown that these women—like many
other immigrant and minority women—are likely to remain in unhappy
or destructive relationships because they are financially dependent and
don't see any way out of their misery.

What these findings should tell caregivers is that we need to be aware
of the cultural differences among our patient population and remain attuned to the psychosocial issues they may be coping with in addition to
their physiological problems so that we are able to treat them accordingly.

I saw this need firsthand when I treated Rosa, a young woman of
Mexican descent who had immigrated to Canada as a young child with
her mother and eight siblings after her parents separated. Life in her
new country hadn't been easy. Her mother had to work very hard just to
support the family and didn't have much time or energy left over to de-
vote to the emotional care and nurturing of her children.

Now, as a young adult, Rosa was still carrying the wounds left by her
difficult childhood. She had never really become assimilated into her
new country. Having married a man of Eastern European descent who
was much more acculturated, she now felt alienated not only from the
local Mexican population but also from her own family, despite having
several brothers and sisters nearby. Her husband, Peter, didn't want to
have anything to do with her family, refusing to visit them even on holi-
days or special occasions. And so when Rosa became anemic and com-
plained of being "tired all the time" during her pregnancy, rather than
urging her to seek the support of her own family, Peter invited *his*
mother to come over from Europe and help out.

Once her anemia was treated successfully, Rosa's family physician re-ferred her to me because she was still feeling excessively fatigued, and he had diagnosed her by a process of elimination as suffering from depres-sion. When she and her husband arrived for her initial appointment, the tension between them was palpable. As her pregnancy progressed, Rosa had become increasingly sad and lonely, and Peter simply couldn't understand or sympathize with her growing feelings of isolation, which were actually being compounded by her having to cope with the so-called help of an overbearing mother-in-law who was, in reality, a stranger to her. The sadder she grew, the more irritated and sullen Peter became, and Rosa, for her part, found it impossible to explain to him what she was feeling. She certainly couldn't discuss the fact that his own mother was part of the problem rather than the solution.

As I spoke with her, it became clear to me that medication alone would not be enough to resolve this young woman's suffering and that an essential part of my treatment would have to be finding a way for Rosa to reassociate with people of her own culture. To do that, I helped her connect with a group of churchgoers who were of Mexican descent so that she would have the support of people among whom she could feel more secure.

Isolation, alienation, and lack of connection can both contribute and surface as symptoms of depression and can, in effect, become a kind of vicious cycle—the more isolated one feels, the more depressed one becomes, and then the depression itself feeds that sense of isolation. For a pregnant woman in a foreign culture, that sense of alienation can be terribly intense, as I've seen for myself again and again among immi-grant populations in Vancouver.

During the 1990s a large number of Hong Kong Chinese immigrated to Canada. Because many of the men continued to work in Hong Kong, their young wives and children lived in a kind of splendid isolation in Canada. Their homes were large and luxurious, but their lives were lonely and sad. Their inability to speak the language would have made it diffi-cult for them to communicate their feelings even if they had been will-ing to seek therapy. To compound the problem, however, they were, for the most part, unable even to fathom what it meant to be depressed, and they were often unwilling to accept medical treatment because of the cultural stigma attached to the very idea of psychiatric illness.

Even for those with husbands who had lived in Canada for some time, the struggle to assimilate and communicate could be overwhelming. Karen, a patient of mine, was one for whom pregnancy was simply one more burden than she could possibly bear. Her husband, a computer programmer, had been born in Canada, and they met when he was on vacation in Hong Kong. After they married, she returned with him to Vancouver, where he expected her to learn English, go out to work, and, in effect, "become Canadian" as quickly as possible. He had never considered, and in fact simply could not comprehend, the difficulties she encountered trying to begin a new life with a new husband in a new country. The harder she struggled, the more irritated he became, and the growing tension between them just added to her stress. She certainly hadn't planned on becoming pregnant, and when she did, it shook her to the core. She was totally unprepared for motherhood and found it impossible to face the many weeks of her pregnancy in a place that was still totally foreign to her and where she felt she had no support at all, even from her husband.

In the end, Karen chose to return to Hong Kong, where she would feel safe within the framework of her family and community. There she gave birth to a healthy baby and also sought treatment for her depression. When she eventually returned to Canada with her newborn, she also brought her mother, who stayed for six months until Karen was finally able to acquire the confidence she needed to thrive on her own and accept both the joys and the responsibilities of motherhood.

Karen was, in the end, one of the lucky ones. She had the resources not only to return to her place of birth but also to bring her mother back to her new country when she needed her. But there are thousands of others who do not have those resources and who therefore must struggle on their own.

To compound the problem, in many immigrant cultures, especially those from developing countries, woman are considered subordinate and are expected to be subservient and obedient to men, including—perhaps particularly—their fathers and their husbands, who often cannot and do not consider it necessary or important to be sensitive to women's feelings. Both Rosa's and Karen's husbands, for example, became irritated and annoyed by their wives' inability to cope with the stresses of marriage, pregnancy, and acculturation simultaneously, and this was even more of an issue for another of my patients. Sonal had come from India as the bride of a man she'd never met. Like the brides of many such arranged marriages, she came from a small agricultural village where she'd had very little education, and she spoke no English.

Sonal came to my office twenty weeks pregnant and gripped by a deep depression. Not only was she pregnant by a man who was still a virtual stranger to her, but she herself was also a stranger in a strange land. As her pregnancy progressed, her depression had deepened, and her husband, who was totally baffled by what was happening to her, felt that he had somehow been tricked into this unhappy marriage and was now talking about divorce.

Because in her culture it was expected that once a woman married she would be happy, raise a family, and simply carry on, Sonal was embarrassed that her marriage of less than a year was falling apart, and she was terrified of having to go back a failure to a place where the future for a divorced woman would be dismal at best. Even in the depths of her depression, Sonal knew that she would be damned either way—whether she stayed in her new country or returned to her native village.

While Karen's story had a happy ending, Sonal's unfortunately did not. Shortly after the birth of their child, her husband filed for divorce, and Sonal was left struggling to adapt to her new culture, raise a child as a single parent, and understand how her life could have gone so wrong. Thankfully, five years later, her family doctor tells me that she is gainfully employed, is caring for her child, and has, in effect, never looked back.

In each of the stories I've just told, it was the husband who was the more acclimated and the wife who was struggling to fit in to her new culture. But that is not always the case. Fatima, for example, was an Afghan woman who'd been granted immigrant status and thrived in her new country. She'd completed her higher education and was teaching at a local community college when she met and married a man who, while he came from her own culture, was not her intellectual equal. Sadly (but perhaps not surprisingly), rather than supporting her emotionally and applauding her successes, this man saw Fatima's every triumph as a threat to his own ego and an insult to his masculinity.

Shortly after becoming pregnant, she discovered that her husband was having an affair with their next-door neighbor, and when she confronted him with his infidelity, all he had to say was "I might as well live with a real Canadian instead of a converted Afghan woman." With that, her world fell apart.

Clearly, Fatima was acculturated only to a point. While she flourished intellectually and had become financially independent, when it came to finding a life partner, she had returned to her cultural roots— and was, unfortunately, left to suffer the emotional and psychological consequences of her all-too-understandable mistake.

The stories of these immigrant women, while certainly unique to their particular situations and cultures, also have relevance for other minority populations and are not so different from what—as we've seen— researchers have learned about Hispanic and African American women in the United States, whose rates of depression were also found to increase in inverse proportion to their perceived sense of well-being.

No One Is Immune

While so far we've looked specifically at women whose cultural alienation and/or economic disadvantage contributed to the stress that led to their antenatal depression, I don't want to give the false impression that women who are educated, are financially stable, and belong to the middle-class majority are somehow immune from this disease. Although that may be the currently accepted belief, I have found—as I mentioned earlier—that women who have been brought up and taught to believe that they can achieve anything they set out to do, that independence is a quality to be valued, and that nothing is beyond their grasp may, when they become pregnant, be carrying a heavy burden of their own.

These women are expected not only to take pregnancy in stride and continue to carry on with whatever their normal activities had been— going to work, caring for the house, preparing the meals—but also to make sure they look good and stay fit both physically and mentally. Having a baby is, in effect, just one more thing a woman like this needs to add to her already long to-do list, and most likely it is expected that she will accomplish the "task" of childbearing without much community support. In our modern urbanized society, most of us are lucky if we even know the names of our next-door neighbors. We're all so involved in simply getting through what we need to do each day that we don't have the time or the inclination even to consider what the virtual stranger in the next house, the next apartment, or the next office might be feeling or needing.

All this is to say that even a happy and well-adjusted pregnant woman, who is content with her life and in her marriage, who has planned her pregnancy and is looking forward to motherhood, may begin to experience feelings of doubt, sadness, and isolation she doesn't understand. She may attribute these feelings to being tired, to her long commute to work, and to long hours at the office that are followed by grocery shopping on the way home and preparing the evening meal before she is finally able to drop, exhausted, into bed, only to do the whole thing again the next day.

She may realize that she's not feeling like herself, that she isn't enjoying the new maternity clothes she's just bought, or that she's no longer so eagerly looking forward to this baby she and her husband had been so excited to conceive. If she's never been depressed before, she may not know why she's feeling this way, and she may be embarrassed by what she considers an inappropriate response to what should be a blissful time in her life. But even if she does recognize her symptoms for what they are, she may be unable to do anything about them, which is also a symptom of depression.

She may, in passing, discuss what she's feeling with her husband, who, despite his own busy schedule, offers to relieve some of the burden by doing the laundry for her. But even so, as she continues to feel worse and worse, she may no longer have the energy required just to prepare the healthy meals she knows she should be eating to nourish herself and the baby she is carrying. As her husband begins to realize that if he doesn't do the cooking there won't be any dinner on the table, he may then take on that task as well. And as the situation goes from bad to worse, she may be unable even to summon up the energy to get out of bed and go to work. Her crying spells may become more frequent, and she may become even less able to cope with the depth of her sadness. At that point she and her husband, often without even knowing it, may be totally engulfed in the emotional maelstrom of her depression.

As I have said, antenatal depression is an equal-opportunity illness. While social isolation, economic deprivation, and unsupportive or destructive relationships surely put some women more at risk than others, it is a dark pit that any woman may fall into no matter what her socioeconomic situation. Pregnancy itself, far from being protective against psychiatric illness, as many continue to believe, can actually *trigger* depression for the first time, exacerbate an already existing condition, or cause the relapse of a depression that had previously been under control.

When Depression Hides in Plain Sight

Marjorie Klein and her colleagues at the Wisconsin Psychiatric Institute have speculated that because there are so many symptoms of depression that mimic symptoms of pregnancy, the statistics reported by studies of depression in women of childbearing age could easily be skewed in one direction or the other.

During their first trimester, many women lose their appetite, while others may experience an excessive desire for particular foods. Most women also feel extremely fatigued and find themselves taking frequent naps even though they might never have done so before. A lot of women are nauseated and simply don't feel well much of the time, and still others complain of feeling "fuzzy in the head" and losing concentration because of the hormonal changes they're experiencing. They might also lose interest in sex, complain of feeling fat, or simply begin to cry for no apparent reason. *But any of these normal signs of pregnancy could also be symptoms of depression.*

Some depressed women lose all interest in eating, while others crave carbohydrates or other specific foods. Many claim to be so tired that they have no energy and simply can't get out of bed. And very often depression is accompanied by an inability to focus or concentrate as well as by an overwhelming feeling of sadness or uncontrolled crying.

Other, less common symptoms that could be attributed to depression include feelings of guilt or of worthlessness and even occasionally the desire to harm oneself.

When Marta became pregnant for the first time, she and her husband, Ethan, were so thrilled that they couldn't wait to share the news with their family and friends. All seemed to be going beautifully until suddenly Marta's mood began to fluctuate wildly for no apparent reason. She might, for example, burst into tears and run from the room when they had visitors, and her baffled husband could only assume that this was "normal" behavior during pregnancy. It wasn't until he described her behavior to another of the husbands during one of their prenatal classes and asked if his wife was also "acting crazy" that Ethan began to realize Marta's mood swings were anything but normal, at which point he urged her to discuss her emotional problems with her obstetrician. But, for whatever reason—perhaps because she was embarrassed to be feeling so sad at a time when she knew she was "supposed" to be joyously anticipating the birth of her baby—two more visits went by without her being able to bring herself to share her state of emotional upheaval. Finally, Ethan decided to accompany Marta and talk to the doctor himself. When her obstetrician, after listening to Ethan's description of her wildly erratic behavior, diagnosed Marta as suffering from antenatal depression, it was almost a relief to both of them to know that there was actually an explanation for what she was experiencing.

In the second trimester most women feel physically well. The baby has started to kick, their pregnancy is starting to show, and they're probably receiving congratulations from friends and colleagues. While many women are reluctant to share their happy news during the first few months lest anything go wrong, by now they are normally confident and feeling good about themselves. The knowledge that they will be bringing a new life into the world is a tremendous boost to their sense of self-worth.

In fact, we used to believe that depression was least prevalent during the second trimester, and fluctuations in mood throughout the three trimesters were seen as an inverted U, with most women feeling "wonderful" during the middle three months of their pregnancy. Now, however, we know that women are vulnerable throughout their pregnancy. If a woman enters her second trimester and begins to have intrusive negative or frightening thoughts, if she feels burdened rather than uplifted by her pregnancy, she should be particularly aware that while her physical health may be fine, there is something very wrong emotionally and she needs to seek help.

By the third trimester the symptoms of pregnancy and depression once more begin to overlap. Many women have gained a considerable amount of weight and retain water that causes swelling of the ankles and fingers. In addition to being breathless and tired simply from dragging themselves around, they may be unable to get comfortable and sleep well at night. At this point they may describe themselves as looking like a "beached whale" and simply can't wait to "get this baby out." *But weight gain, fatigue, sleeplessness, poor self-image, and negative ideations are also symptoms of depression.* Thus women need to be aware of the point at which their normal feelings are so dark and relentless as to have crossed the bounds of normalcy.

Linda, for example, was a social worker who, in the course of her work, sometimes had to remove babies from mothers who were unable or unwilling to care for them. Although she enjoyed most aspects of her job, this was one that she dreaded—so much so, in fact, that she and her husband had decided she should leave social work and seek a different career. Before that could happen, however, Linda became pregnant herself, and by her third trimester she was in the throes of a major depression.

She was beginning to conjure up vivid mental images of all the women she'd caused to lose their babies during her years as a social worker. Then she began to imagine that someone from her office would discover she was depressed and take away her baby as soon as it was born. So real-seeming was this delusion that when she finally did give birth, Linda kept it a secret from her colleagues; even her family members were allowed to visit for no more than a few minutes, and only one at a time. Only after receiving rigorous treatment combining two medications—one for her depression, the other for her delusions—and intense therapy with a psychologist did she recover from her illness and seek a new career that would be less burdensome emotionally and psychologically.

Linda's stress and guilt about having to cause pain to other women by removing at-risk babies from their homes clearly contributed during her own pregnancy to severe depression with psychotic ideation. Her story, however, should be taken as a cautionary tale for any woman who experiences such unrealistic thought patterns. If she begins to think she'd be willing to do almost anything just to be "free" of her pregnancy, if she becomes obsessed with dwelling on the health of her baby, if she looks "hideous" to herself every time she glances in the mirror, or if she is running to the doctor between scheduled appointments because of some perceived physical problem, she needs to understand that these may be signals of depression.

One reason for my writing this book is to let every woman know that if she is feeling unbearably sad, guilty, or hopeless at *any* point during her pregnancy, these *are not* normal feelings, and she needs to address them as surely and swiftly as she would a rise in blood pressure or unusual staining or cramping. Just as she wouldn't endanger herself or her baby by waiting until her high blood pressure turned into preeclampsia or the cramping led to preterm delivery, she must not wait until her symptoms of depression become so severe that they threaten not only her own well-being but also that of the child she is carrying. As we'll be discussing further in the chapters that follow, psychological and emotional stress can ultimately be just as dangerous to both mother and child as any physical complication.

One woman who came into my practice was astute and alert enough to recognize those feelings in herself early on, but even so, she had a hard time convincing anyone else. "Dr. Misri," Anita lamented when she arrived for her first appointment, "I have tried and tried to convince people I'm depressed, but no one will believe me! It seems as if I have to be my own psychiatrist and diagnose myself!" Sad to say, Anita wasn't really wrong about that.

Because she was such a strong woman, the one upon whom her family and friends were used to depending for guidance and support, no one wanted to think that Anita could be depressed, and when she tried to convey to them what she was feeling, they just told her that she "couldn't afford to be depressed." No doubt they truly found it difficult to believe that someone like Anita would become depressed "just because" she was pregnant, but it's probably also true that *they* "couldn't afford" to think of her as depressed.

Anita, nevertheless, knew she was depressed for the very reason that she was having feelings she'd never experienced before. When she came to me she was thirty-nine years old and twenty-one weeks pregnant. But, she told me, she'd actually recognized her depression eighteen weeks before—when her pregnancy was only in its third week.

Anita had suffered a miscarriage when she was in her early twenties and had been trying to become pregnant again ever since. The hallmark of her particular depression was an extraordinary preoccupation with her pregnancy and the well-being of the baby she was carrying—feelings that might not be considered unusual for a woman in her situation. But Anita knew that her awakening over and over again during the night worrying about whether her baby was developing normally went way beyond the bounds of normalcy. Luckily, her astute interpretation of her own symptoms brought her into treatment when it was still early enough to intervene and make sure that the remainder of her pregnancy went smoothly, with no worsening of her condition.

But why is it that a perfectly normal woman who has never before experienced a depressive episode would suddenly be afflicted during pregnancy? That's a very good question with any number of possible answers. It could be a physiological reaction to the hormonal changes attendant on pregnancy. It could be a reaction to the stress of adding pregnancy to an already overloaded to-do list. It could be triggered by the resurfacing of a previous unresolved trauma that had lain dormant on an unconscious level for years. Or it could be a combination of physiological and psychological factors, including a genetic component.

When Depression Strikes for the First Time

For a woman who has not previously experienced a serious depression, the first onset during pregnancy can strike without warning, and because pregnancy-triggered depression has been so little studied and so unpublicized or not discussed, it is likely to go unrecognized by the woman's physician as well as the woman herself, whatever her level of education and sophistication.

While women these days worry about all sorts of behaviors that might hurt their baby, from drinking alcohol to taking medications to such seemingly innocuous activities as having a manicure or sitting in a hot tub—and there are even Web sites on which these bits of information (or misinformation) are exchanged—the last thing on most women's minds when they become pregnant is worrying that they will become depressed. So if depression does strike, they may very well dismiss their symptoms as those that occur normally during pregnancy.

When Depression Deepens

If a woman has not previously been depressed, its onset during pregnancy can, as I've said, hit her like a bolt from the blue. That is understandable. What's less easy to comprehend, however, is why so many women who are already suffering symptoms of depression seem to believe that their illness will be "cured" by pregnancy.

If a woman is prone to thyroid problems, it is safe to assume that she wouldn't expect her pregnancy to alleviate that preexisting condition; on the contrary, she would alert her obstetrician so that the doctor would be aware of the need to monitor it closely and treat it accordingly. Yet a lot of women apparently cling to the notion that pregnancy will somehow magically fix their depression—just as many rely on having a child as a way to fix a troubled marriage. By now, however, we should all be aware that if a marriage is in trouble, a baby isn't going to fix it. On the contrary, the baby is more likely to become the third angle in a dysfunctional relationship triangle. And pregnancy is even less likely to fix a depression (or any other psychological problem, for that matter). In fact, the hormonal changes that pregnancy brings with it will, more than likely, exacerbate an already existing depression.

Juliana was depressed during her first pregnancy but had done very well with group and individual therapy and did not require medication. After the birth of her baby, however, her depression deepened, and in addition she began to experience symptoms of generalized anxiety disorder. But because she wanted to breast-feed, she was reluctant to take antidepressants. (I'll be discussing the issue of breast-feeding and antidepressant medication in Chapter 9.) As a result, her condition continued to deteriorate until, finally, she agreed to begin treatment with Zoloft. After that, she did start to feel better, but she continued to struggle with residual symptoms of generalized anxiety. Then, knowing full well that her condition was not completely stabilized, she decided to become pregnant again.

By the time I met her, Juliana was already anxious and depressed, and she finally confessed to me that she had unilaterally decided to discontinue her pharmacological treatment. Thankfully, once she was back on the medication her condition stabilized, and with careful monitoring and adjustment of dosages, she was able to deliver a healthy baby with absolutely no complications.

The Motherisk Program, based in Toronto, advises expectant mothers about the potential risk of fetal exposure to drugs, chemicals, radiation, and other toxic substances. An article published in 2001 by Adrienne Einarson and her Motherisk group points to the dangers of discontinuing antidepressant medications during pregnancy. The researchers studied thirty-six pregnant women, thirty-three of whom had abruptly discontinued their medications and three who had gone off them gradually because of their fear of birth defects. Almost a third of those in the study reported that they had actually contemplated suicide because the physical and psychological symptoms they experienced were so severe as to seem unbearable, and four of them required hospitalization. Luckily, once they'd received counseling, twenty-two of these women resumed their medication and were thus able to manage their depression and deliver healthy babies. Four others no longer required medication, but the outcomes of the remaining ten, who did not resume treatment, are unknown.

In the nonpregnant population 40 to 60 percent of patients who discontinue their medication prematurely will experience a relapse. Among pregnant women with recurrent major depression, 75 percent will relapse, and among those, 69 percent will relapse during the first trimester.

It is generally accepted by the psychiatric community that once antidepressant medication is begun, the treatment should continue for at least twelve months to ensure remission and prevent relapse, and it's important to understand that the same guidelines should be followed for pregnant women. In fact, because pregnancy itself puts women at greater risk for relapse, it may be even more important for them to continue medication than it would be for those who are not pregnant—a recommendation that is consistent with the Expert Consensus Guidelines on Treatment of Depression in Women, formulated in 2001.

Not so many years ago most doctors would have taken the opposite approach. Typically, a woman would discontinue her medication as soon as she discovered she'd conceived, and we, as health care providers, would recommend that she resume taking her medications after she'd given birth. Now, largely as a result of studies, we have much better information about the risk/benefit ratios of a woman's remaining on medication during pregnancy. Yet I still meet some physicians who, because of what I can only assume is their own bias or lack of knowledge, continue to encourage their patients to go through pregnancy unmedicated.

Just this past year, when I was speaking at a seminar to a group of women doctors about the use of medication during pregnancy and lactation, I met one family physician who explained to me that she saw her patients through pregnancy with only what she called "weekly counseling." Since I had admitted one of her patients to my hospital just the week before because she'd become increasingly suicidal, I had a difficult time containing my frustration at such a misguided approach, particularly from a female colleague with a large obstetrical practice. When I asked her whether her patients relapsed and, if they did, how she treated them, her answer was simply "I humor them along until the baby comes, and then I put them on medication post-partum." I have to admit that in that moment I felt totally defeated, as if everything I'd been trying to say, not only to the group of women I'd just addressed but to all the medical students, residents, and family practitioners I'd been working so hard to educate, had fallen on deaf ears.

Aisha is a perfect example of the adverse consequences I *know* can result when a pregnant woman, usually with the best of intentions, decides to stop taking her meds. After several depressive episodes, Aisha had been stabilized on Effexor XR for about four years when she and her health care provider jointly decided to discontinue it once she became pregnant. Predictably, Aisha relapsed within four weeks, and by her third trimester she was so severely depressed that she had to be admitted to the hospital, where her medications were reinstated. At that point, however, her previous dose was no longer effective and had to be increased in order for her to achieve remission.

When I met with him, Aisha's husband blamed himself along with all the well-meaning friends and relatives who, he said, had "badgered" her into giving up her medication "for the sake of the baby." Now not only was she having to suffer the pain of a serious depression and the trauma of hospitalization, but she was, in fact, exposing her unborn child to even higher levels of the medication she'd been trying to avoid as well as to the stresses attendant upon her depression—a subject I'll be addressing specifically in Chapter 11.

My point here is that even though no woman would knowingly subject her baby to any toxic or potentially damaging substance, some women don't really have a choice. If they are taking antidepressant medication at the time they decide to conceive (assuming the pregnancy is wanted and planned), *they need to continue their medication in order to remain stable throughout the pregnancy.*

Aisha's child is now six years old, and I still receive Christmas cards from Aisha thanking me for "saving her life." In retrospect, she realizes what a terrible mistake it was for her to discontinue her medication and become pregnant while she was in the midst of a depressive relapse, yet time and again I see women in my practice who want to rush into pregnancy despite my telling them that doing so will almost surely be detrimental to their emotional health. And for every reason I give for delaying their pregnancy, they have an excuse for doing the opposite: "But I love children," "But I've already waited so long." I know I shouldn't be surprised. After all these years I certainly shouldn't be shocked. Yet I do still wonder at the thought process that leads these women to take on the added responsibility of childbearing at a time when their own mental health is so fragile.

Sally came to me, accompanied by her mother, for a prepregnancy consultation because she was going to be married in two months. At twenty-seven, Sally had already been suffering from depression and taking medication for fourteen years—since she was just thirteen. By the time she entered college at the age of nineteen, one medication was no longer enough to control her illness, and when I met her she was taking both Celexa, an antidepressant, and lithium, a mood stabilizer. Despite the medications, however, Sally was once more starting to experience fluctuations of mood. Because of the stress of planning and anticipating her forthcoming wedding, she was feeling anxious and not sleeping very well.

Although Sally had ostensibly come to consult with me about whether or not it would be "safe" for her to have a baby, when I counseled her to wait at least six months after the wedding to be sure her mood was stabilized, it was clear that Sally really didn't want my advice. What she wanted was a baby. In fact, she said, she'd wanted a child ever since she was a teenager. Becoming a mother was her ultimate goal, and to her waiting six months would be nothing but more wasted time. She felt she'd already waited long enough.

Her own mother had returned to work when Sally was just six weeks old, and Sally, who clearly harbored negative feelings about her mother's choice, was determined to give her own child the "perfect" life she felt she'd never had. But she was in such a hurry to get started that she simply couldn't see the wisdom of waiting. She couldn't see that her chances of becoming the perfect mother she wanted to be would improve greatly once her own emotions were under control.

The next time I saw her, six months later, Sally was eleven weeks pregnant and obviously seriously depressed. Her whole demeanor broadcast the fact that she was feeling hopeless and defeated. Once more she was accompanied by her mother, whose anger at her defensive daughter was all too visible on her face.

There are many lessons to be learned from Sally's sad story. The first and most important of these is that the timing of a pregnancy must be right—both your body and your mind must be prepared. This is truly a fact of nature that becomes clear when we look to the animal kingdom. For most animals, as well as fish and birds, there is a mating season and certain rituals related to preparing for procreation. Birds migrate from all over the world to meet and mate; salmon swim upstream; mammals come into season at particular times of year. And for a human being with a depressive illness who is constantly struggling to balance the sensitive neurotransmitters that control mood swings, that timing is all the more important.

The second lesson is to be certain you're becoming pregnant for the right reasons. Understand that you can't use a child to right a perceived wrong from your own past, particularly if you haven't come to terms with or resolved the experience for yourself. And the third is that when you do decide to conceive, you need to have the complete support of your health care providers, your family, and, most important of all, your partner.

After Sally's first appointment, I made certain that when she returned she'd be accompanied by her husband so that together we could formulate a plan for managing her depression—and help her finally to understand that after having this baby, it would be best if she waited before she became pregnant again. Unbelievably, in the midst of her depression, while she was still carrying her first child, Sally was already talking about having another!

For any woman with a history of depression, even if she is taking medication and her condition is stabilized, there is a strong probability that the condition will worsen with pregnancy.

In my own hospital, we have followed the cases of thirty-six pregnant women whose depression was being controlled and stabilized with medication. During the initial phase of the study, which was funded by a grant from the Vancouver Foundation, we tracked their progress throughout pregnancy and for eight months postpartum. Since then, we have received a second grant that is allowing us to follow them and their babies for an additional four years. The criteria for their inclusion were that they had to be depressed while pregnant, that they were between eight and thirty-three weeks of gestation when they entered the study, and that they were not abusing over-the-counter medications and were substance-free aside from their antidepressant medication.

Because of the length and depth of the study, we were able to collect a great deal of important information, including the effects of medication on the fetus and the possible risks of breast-feeding while taking antidepressant drugs—both subjects that will be addressed later in this book. The point I want to make here, however, is that almost one-third of the women in our study experienced an exacerbation of their depression during pregnancy that required adjustments to their levels of medication. Yet many health care providers continue to remain unaware of the link between pregnancy and the worsening of depression. For that reason alone, I can't stress enough the need for any woman who is being treated for or has previously experienced a depressive episode to be aware of and monitor her own condition. It is, in fact, imperative that she be an astute observer of her own mood and proactive about communicating any perceived emotional change to her doctor.

Doctors may not be attuned to the need for monitoring their patients' moods, or they may be too hurried to take the time to do what is necessary, but no woman should be too busy to pay attention to her emotional and mental health. Even if, to her, depression seems to be a thing of the past, she needs to understand that pregnancy may be the trigger that causes it to reappear.

When Depression Returns

Women such as Sally and those whose cases were followed in my hospital knew at the time they became pregnant that while their depressive symptoms might be under control, their illness was not "cured." It was not a thing of the past. But any past history of depression, even if it occurred only once and many years before, still puts women at risk for a recurrence during pregnancy.

Dina and her sister Lisa, for example, had both suffered bouts of depression during their teenage years and had been treated successfully without medication. By pure chance, the two sisters married brothers whom they'd met separately without even being aware they were related. Both were happy in their marriages and planned their pregnancies with much cheerful anticipation of motherhood.

At about twenty-six weeks into her pregnancy, however, Dina became increasingly irritable and moody. Her husband, who was upset and confused because he had no idea what was happening to his wife, confided in his brother, who then informed him that Lisa, too, had suffered from a mild depression during her pregnancy but had recognized her symptoms early on and been treated successfully with interpersonal therapy. Unfortunately, Dina didn't realize soon enough that her change in mood was, in fact, a recurrence of her previous depression, so it wasn't until her husband spoke to his brother about it that the family history she shared with her sister came to light.

Dina's story illustrates the need for *any* woman who has suffered a depressive episode at any time in her life to be aware that she is at risk for a recurrence during pregnancy and to report any perceived changes in her mood to her health care provider.

Knowledge Is Power

Individual health care providers—again, I must stress, with the best of intentions—may either miss or misinterpret even the most obvious signs of depression, or may allow their own biases regarding the use of medication during pregnancy to color or guide their treatment recommendations. For these reasons, I believe that every woman must do all she can to educate herself.

Over and over again we hear about patients' need to advocate for themselves, to find out all they can about their condition, and to seek second opinions. In no case is this advice more important than it is for a woman who knows better than anyone else what she is experiencing mentally and emotionally and who needs to make decisions for herself.

Those decisions ought to be based on hard medical and scientific evidence about the potential risks of taking medication during pregnancy versus the risks (to both the woman and her baby) of her lapsing or relapsing into the painful pit of depression.

To help every woman do that, in the chapters that follow I'll be discussing additional factors that are likely to exacerbate or complicate antenatal depression as well as what research has to tell us about the risk/benefit ratio of taking antidepressant medication.

5

Compounding the Risk

In the previous chapter we touched on some of the psychosocial stressors that are likely to put certain women more at risk than others for depression during pregnancy. Women whose marriages are already unstable, women who have been subjected to present or past emotional or physical violence or abuse, and those who lack strong social support are, as we have seen, those most likely to find the additional stress of a pregnancy "too much" and, therefore, to become depressed—if they weren't already. While it would be easy to dismiss these particular risk factors as belonging to those who are disadvantaged socially, economically, or educationally, and to assume that if a woman doesn't fall into one of these categories she is immune, I cannot emphasize strongly enough that disharmony, abuse, and social alienation do not so nicely discriminate among their victims.

Social alienation, as I've said, is endemic to the rush and crush of daily life in a world where even television commercials show little girls checking their PDAs with their parents to coordinate schedules. And unless the occupants are celebrities whose every private moment and personal peccadillo is subject to coverage in the tabloids, no one can really know what goes on behind the closed doors of even the most affluent homes or apartments. In fact, when people in high-powered jobs have to make multiple important, often difficult decisions every day, they may take their pent-up stress and anxiety home, where it is inappropriately released on the most available person, generally a partner or spouse.

Marital Disharmony, Violence, and Depression: A Tragic Triangle

As I mentioned earlier, there are still a number of people around who seem to believe that having a baby is the answer to fixing the marital discord. In fact, in my practice I've treated many, many women who mistakenly thought that their pregnancy would be the cure-all not only for their depression but also for their unhappy home life. How tragically wrong they were!

It's not difficult to understand why a troubled marriage would lead anyone to feel depressed. Most people embark upon marriage assuming that it will be happy and fulfilling for both partners. When this does not happen—or when the happiness isn't reciprocated—the blow to one's self-esteem can be devastating. If you then add to that situation the additional stress of bringing a new life into the unhappy home, more often than not you've created a formula for disaster. Pregnancy is a time when women need unconditional support from those who are closest to them. They crave attention and require their partners to validate the emotional and physical changes they are experiencing because the hormonal changes going on in their bodies make them particularly sensitive in pregnancy.

In one study done by Dr. Richard Johanson in the United Kingdom, each of 417 women entering the hospital for delivery was given a self-rating scale for depression and another for marital disharmony. When the results were tallied, they revealed a significant association between those who had experienced antenatal depression and those who were having marital difficulties. Perhaps even more significantly, however, only a small proportion of these women had been found to be depressed when previously interviewed by their family physicians.

One possible reason for this could be that the family doctor simply failed to diagnose their depression. But it might also be that when there is disharmony in a marriage, it can trigger antenatal depression even if the woman was not previously depressed. Conversely, if the marriage isn't totally stable and supportive, the onset of depression during pregnancy can trigger even greater disharmony.

Increased irritability is one of the behaviors most often associated with depression, and although it may be simply the outward manifestation of inner sadness, the depressed woman's husband or partner—particularly if she has not previously been depressed or if he is unaware of the many ways depression can manifest—is likely to see only her anger and irritability, not the underlying sadness. Because he is probably the person closest to her, he is also the one most likely to bear the brunt of her harsh words or short temper. Unless he is extremely supportive and understanding, he may see himself as the innocent victim of a woman who has suddenly "gone nuts." However he reacts, be it holding his tongue or lashing back in anger, any preexisting, smoldering marital tension is likely to become inflamed as the woman's pregnancy proceeds and her depression deepens.

The husband of one of my patients actually moved out of the house during the third trimester of her pregnancy because he could no longer cope with coming home every day to what he later described to me as an "emotional hurricane." Luckily, once both he and his wife understood that her radical personality transformation was a symptom of depression rather than a normal aspect of pregnancy, he was able to put his own feelings aside in order to support her, and he subsequently moved back in.

If marital discord increases a woman's risk for antenatal depression, actual abuse or physical violence creates a situation that can explode into an emotional tsunami during pregnancy. One study conducted by Dr. Donna Stewart at the University of Toronto found that when there is violence in a relationship, it is likely to escalate alarmingly during pregnancy. According to Dr. Stewart, the rate of physical abuse among pregnant women in diverse areas across North America ranges from 4 to 20 percent. Among the general population, one in every six women in

Canada and 2.5 million women in the United States are abused. My own patients have actually reported being kicked in the stomach during pregnancy. as if their abusers were trying to hurt not only them but also the babies they were carrying. As horrifying as I find this, I also know that abusers are not restricted to any one culture or socioeconomic group, but can be hiding behind the door of any typical middle-class home.

And what about the women who are being abused? They are often as beaten down mentally as they are physically battered and bruised, and because they are depressed, feel hopeless. and are totally lacking in self-esteem, they are unlikely to see any way out—particularly when they are about to have a baby and may, therefore, feel more dependent financially on their partner and believe that they won't be able to survive on their own with a new baby. They don't report the violence because they believe it is somehow their fault and that they will be blamed for what's happening to them if anyone else, including their health care provider, finds out. The onus, therefore, falls on the health care provider to try to ferret out the information in a way that will allow the woman to confide in him or her. Too often. I think, we suspect that all is not well in the home but are nevertheless reluctant to ask the necessary questions. I can't stress strongly enough the health care provider's *need* to ask these questions and abused women's *need* to confide in their doctors so that together they can prevent the kind of terrible tragedy that befell one of my patients.

Reesa came to see me when she was about seven months pregnant. Although she had a history of depression. her symptoms were presently in remission. Like many teenagers, she had abused drugs to help alleviate her depression, but she assured me that she'd been clean throughout her pregnancy. What she didn't tell me, however, was that her partner, Jack, whom she'd met at a Narcotics Anonymous meeting just eight months earlier, was still using narcotics in the form of prescription pain-killers.

Since Reesa's depression and drug abuse made hers a high-risk pregnancy, we asked (as we do routinely in such cases) that she and Jack come in together for a prenatal assessment. When I met Jack, I had a strong gut feeling that he could be violent. I didn't ask him directly if he was abusing Reesa, but I did manage to discover, through cautious questioning, that he was still struggling with drugs.

It was not, however, until her final antenatal visit that Reesa described to me the physical violence to which she'd been regularly subjected throughout her pregnancy. At that point, I alerted the appropriate child welfare agency so that they would be able to monitor the situation, but even so, just eight weeks after she gave birth, I received a telephone call informing me that Reesa and the baby had been admitted to the hospital with multiple injuries.

Thankfully, both Reesa and her baby recovered from their physical injuries. The baby was put into foster care, and Reesa now visits with her frequently, trying to form a bond in anticipation of the day when, she hopes, her daughter will be returned to her. But it was not until her situation was out in the open that Reesa could bring herself to tell me she'd been scared to death of Jack the entire time she was pregnant.

Although Reesa's case is extreme—in most cases the abuser does not directly attack his own child but confines his violence to attacking his partner or spouse—her inability to seek help or to leave the relationship is not so different from what happens to any woman who is regularly subjected to physical abuse. Living with violence almost inevitably erodes the woman's sense of self, and the longer the violence continues, the less likely it is that she will be able to extricate herself from her untenable situation. Moreover, speaking specifically of the external factors that put women at greater risk of antenatal depression, it should be obvious that domestic violence would be one of the key stressors. And it is also important to understand that even if the abuser does not harm the fetus or the baby directly, research has shown that any child brought into an environment filled with rage, fear, and tension is at great risk for developing serious psychological problems later on.

Mothers Who Lose Mothers: When Support Disappears

Among the reasons marital disharmony and/or abuse increases the risk for depression is the fact that most women in these situations are unwilling or unable to share their pain or have no one to whom they can turn for support. We've already discussed the importance of having strong community and family support during pregnancy, so it stands to reason that this is a time when any woman would turn to her mother for advice and comfort or simply to discuss what's happening to her body. It is also a time when women are likely to think about the way they themselves were mothered and to consider, if they haven't already done so, which of their mother's habits or ways of parenting they want to emulate and which they hope to avoid. If their relationship with their mother was difficult, this may be a time when they want to heal it. If it was good, warm, and close, this is a time when it almost always becomes closer. In fact, women who have a particularly good relationship with their mothers will generally feel particularly good about their own pregnancy. So when a woman loses her mother either during or just prior to pregnancy, that loss can be a trigger for antenatal depression. If their relationship was less than ideal, death robs the woman of the opportunity to reconcile or repair it; if it was especially close, death denies her a key source of support, as it did my patient Amy.

Perhaps because her parents were divorced when she was very young, Amy had always been extremely close to her mother. Even after she was married, they lived in the same city, and when she became pregnant, she shared all her plans as well as every little physical change she was experiencing with her mother. Then, early one morning, she was awakened out of a deep sleep by a phone call informing her that her mother, who was only sixty-two years old and in seemingly good health, had died suddenly of a massive heart attack.

Amy was devastated. It was almost impossible for her to take in the fact that her mother, with whom she'd had a long phone conversation just hours before, planning the colors for the nursery, was now gone. Rushing to her apartment, Amy stared in disbelief at her mother's lifeless body. Instead of making plans for the nursery, she would now be planning a funeral.

Her depression came on suddenly. Instead of thinking about her own impending motherhood, she found herself ruminating incessantly upon her loss and unable to get the picture of her mother's dead body out of her mind. All the joy she'd been feeling was gone; now there was only sorrow and increasingly uncontrolled anxiety.

Anxiety, as I'll be discussing further in Chapter 7, is one of the ways depression frequently manifests in women, and depressive illness marked by anxiety is also likely to show itself when a woman becomes pregnant after being treated for infertility or subsequent to a previous miscarriage. But both infertility and miscarriage can also be accompanied by or trigger depression in women.

When One Can't Conceive: Depression and Infertility

Infertility affects about 15 percent of all women of childbearing age worldwide. Certainly not all of these women will suffer from depression, but among those who are vulnerable, ongoing infertility treatment can trigger a depressive episode. In fact, several studies done over the last few years have shown a strong link between infertility and depressive illness.

One particular study conducted at the School of Public Health in Minneapolis, Minnesota, and published in the *Journal of Psychosomatic Obstetrics and Gynecology* investigated the prevalence of depression among women diagnosed with infertility compared to a control group. The study found that a significantly higher number of women in the infertile group were depressed or had a past history of depression. Interestingly, among those who were depressed, the majority had experienced their first episode just prior to their diagnosis of infertility. Since infertility is defined as being unable to conceive after one year of regular sexual intercourse without contraception, one might speculate that these women had already diagnosed themselves, or feared what the diagnosis would be, before it was confirmed by their doctor.

Yet another study, conducted by B. J. Berg and colleagues, examined 104 infertile couples and found that more than 50 percent of the women in the study experienced psychiatric symptoms, including those of depression. They felt guilty or responsible, suffered from low self-esteem, and in general experienced more disruption of their lives than did their male partners. And an investigation by B. S. Kee and colleagues of 138 Korean women who were receiving infertility treatment, published in the *Journal of Assisted Reproduction and Genetics*, found that they tested higher on the Anxiety Inventory and the Beck Depression Inventory than women who were fertile. Finally, Dr. K. M. Anderson and colleagues in the United Kingdom, who interviewed couples referred to an infertility clinic, also found that the women reported more clinically significant levels of anxiety, a greater impact of infertility on their lives, and less satisfaction with life in general. The women reported that their infertility had impacted their sexuality, were likely to blame themselves, had low self-esteem, and tended to avoid contact with their friends.

What these results indicate is that if a woman is vulnerable to depression, being labeled "childless" can become the sole focus of her life, overriding or negating anything else she may have achieved or any other success she's experienced. These women consider themselves incomplete. They may set aside their career and distance themselves from friends and family because they believe that no one else can understand the gravity of their situation or the pain they are feeling. The more they believe they are misunderstood, the more depressed they become and the more they tend to isolate themselves, intentionally or unintentionally.

How the woman's family and friends react can have a significant impact upon her ability to deal with her situation. A study done in Turkey used a depression inventory scale to compare fifty infertile women with fifty healthy control subjects. What the researchers found was that depression and anxiety occurred more frequently among those in the infertile group who received negative reactions from their husbands, their husbands' families, and their social group.

This can make coping with their situation that much more difficult for women living in societies (mainly in developing countries) or cultures that place a high value on fertility, and where not to bear children causes women to be labeled social outcasts. Clearly, however, any woman who is diagnosed with infertility needs extra nurturing, positive support, and the encouragement of those people to whom she feels most answerable and responsible.

When Natalie came to me she was married for the third time and had been trying to conceive for five years. She was forty years old, and she knew her biological clock was ticking relentlessly. Neither of her first two husbands had wanted a child, and her present marriage was filled with tension because her husband was anxious for them to have children. They'd been to a fertility clinic and found that his sperm count and motility levels were normal, which meant that the "fault" lay with Natalie. As a result, in addition to the stress of infertility, she was suffering the added stress of fearing that she might lose her husband.

After her first failed in vitro fertilization (IVF) cycle, she began to spend sleepless nights ruminating about her inability to conceive but, not unnaturally, decided this was a "normal" response to the initial failure. When the second cycle failed, her ruminations became more severe, as did her guilt and dread of yet a third failed attempt. It was at that point her doctor referred her to me, because he felt that, given her mental state, she would not be an appropriate candidate for the third in vitro treatment. At that point, virtually every waking moment of Natalie's life was preoccupied with dark, intrusive thoughts, and she had become so dysfunctional that she'd had to take a leave of absence from her job. Although she was trying to "keep herself busy" and distract herself from thinking about her infertility, she was finding it increasingly difficult to concentrate.

When I met her husband, it was clear that Natalie's fear of rejection was far from accurate. In fact, he was extremely supportive, but he also explained that he was finding it more and more challenging to communicate with his wife on a rational level. Even though her IVF treatments were on hold, she was still obsessively checking her menstrual calendar and could focus on nothing but having sex at the "best time" for conception. In fact, she had decided that her doctor had given up on her (which was totally untrue) and was determined to "win the infertility war" on her own. While her husband knew that her thinking was completely unrealistic, he also understood that there was absolutely nothing he could do to convince her of this while she was in her present state of mind.

A former dancer and the director of a large dance company, Natalie was a perfectionist who had always succeeded at anything to which she put her mind. Now, for the first time, she was unable to control her own destiny, and she felt "cheated." Although she had a résumé full of impressive titles, the one title she couldn't add (which, of course, became the one most important to her) was that of mother. After our initial interview, Natalie began a course of cognitive behavior therapy (which I'll be explaining in detail in Chapter 10) to help her examine her distorted thought patterns and to address her self-defeating behaviors. Within ten to twelve sessions her intrusive, ruminative thoughts began to dissipate and she was able to appreciate the fact that her obsessive thinking was, in fact, unrealistic and a symptom of her ongoing depression. At that point she was able to resume IVF. Her third treatment, happily, resulted in a successful pregnancy, and as of this writing we are monitoring Natalie's mood to ensure stability in pregnancy and in the postpartum period.

For a woman such as Natalie, who has always known what to do to achieve professional success and who has always felt that her fate was hers to control, infertility may come as a terrible blow to her self-esteem. Not only has her body betrayed her, but for the first time she is unable to fix the problem on her own. When that happens, she may find herself struggling with symptoms of sadness, ruminations on her "failure," and excessive guilt.

When depression and infertility occur simultaneously, one might assume that if the infertility is treated successfully and the woman conceives, her depression will lift, and therefore that it would be more important to treat the infertility than the depression. However, several studies have shown that this is not the case. Infertility treatment can be harsh and invasive. It can take over one's life and put a strain on one's career and one's marriage, and if it continues to be unsuccessful over a period of time, it can lead to even deeper despair. For those reasons, it is important to be certain that the patient is mentally equipped and emotionally strong enough to deal with the treatment itself, as well as with the possibility that it won't succeed. This is particularly true if the woman has had a history of depression and is being maintained on medication. Years ago, there were many fertility clinics that refused to treat women on antidepressant medications, but, mercifully, this unenlightened way of thinking is becoming far less prevalent.

Gina, a patient of mine, was in a long-term same-sex relationship and wanted to become a mother at any cost. Even though she was prone to depression and was taking medication, she was determined to go through as many cycles of IVF as it took to succeed. Her partner, a psychologist, was well aware of the mental and emotional problems attendant on this kind of treatment, and she encouraged Gina to continue her medications during her IVF. As it turned out, after four cycles Gina finally conceived. Thanks to her determination, her inner strength, and her network of support, she went through the process with minimal psychological trauma. I've heard women say they were afraid that their antidepressants might actually reduce or interfere with their chances of conceiving, but this is simply not true. Furthermore, if, as we have already seen, the stress of pregnancy can trigger, deepen, or cause a relapse of depression, the much greater stress of being diagnosed with and enduring the stormy ups and downs of treatment for infertility are all the more likely to be associated with a serious depression.

In addition to the depressive reaction to the diagnosis and the arduous nature of the treatment, however, it is possible that many women are also reacting to the fertility medications themselves. Even if they have begun treatment with a positive attitude, the fertility drugs (Clomid and Pergonal) they are given to produce more eggs, which act on the pituitary gland, may disrupt the stability of mood. Thus the drugs themselves may lead to depressive symptoms including mood swings and sleep disturbance, as well as bloating and headaches, all of which can compound the anxiety created by the infertility. Progesterone, which is prescribed to help maintain the pregnancy once fertilization takes place, can also increase irritability and cause unstable moods.

For all of these reasons, it is vitally important that any woman embarking on infertility treatment be aware of the emotional turmoil this may entail so that she can monitor her own mood and be prepared to seek help if necessary. Finally, if her treatment fails, she must be prepared for that outcome, too. When her identity as an "infertile woman" is confirmed, she may undergo what the Canadian researcher Dr. Jan Rehner has described as a "painful reassembly of self."

Rona, a flight attendant, became a patient of mine when, after several attempts at in vitro fertilization, she finally had to accept the fact that she would be childless. It took two years of therapy before Rona was able to integrate this knowledge into her self-identity and accept herself as worthwhile and "of use" in other ways. In the end, however, she told me that she believed there was a "reason" why she could not become a mother and that she wanted and needed to embark on a path of spiritual exploration. Now she travels to Nepal, Tibet, and remote parts of China at least three months a year, helping people in whatever way she can. She tells me that she always returns home feeling gratified by whatever assistance she was able to provide. She has found a path to fulfillment or "nirvana" beyond motherhood.

When Pregnancy Loss Triggers Depression

If the inability to conceive is associated with the onset of depression, it's no wonder that the loss of a pregnancy would also be reason for women to become depressed. As the pregnancy proceeds, the mother-to-be quite naturally develops an attachment to the baby she is carrying. And now, because of technological advances that have made ultrasound a common way of monitoring pregnancy, most women actually get to "see" their baby developing. By ten weeks of gestation, the expectant mother has generally developed some sort of mental image of the fetus, and by twenty weeks, when the baby starts kicking, this sense of her child as a living being becomes strong indeed. If she subsequently loses that baby, it's as if she had experienced a death, and becoming depressed could therefore be viewed as a natural reaction.

One study found that women who miscarried exhibited markedly elevated symptoms of depression as compared to a control group at two weeks after the miscarriage, while another, completed by M. Beutel and colleagues and published in *Psychosomatic Medicine* in 1995, found that at six and twelve months after pregnancy loss women who had miscarried did not differ from the control group in terms of depression. It appears, then, that a normal reactive depression does lift with the passage of time, as does the grief associated with any loss. But for some women the depression is deeper and more pervasive, requiring professional counseling and treatment.

A woman's risk of becoming depressed after miscarriage as well as the depth of the depression appear to depend on a number of factors: her age, the number of times she has miscarried, whether or not she has other children, her attitude toward the pregnancy, and whether or not she has a prior history of depression.

Claudia Klier and her colleagues in the Department of Psychiatry at the University of Vienna have found that the frequency of miscarriage among women who conceive is approximately 14 percent. Among women ages twenty to twenty-four, however, it is only about 9 percent, increasing to 75 percent for those over forty-five. So in addition to the fact that older women may be at higher risk for depression in any case, those who miscarry bear the added burden of knowing that their chances of conceiving again and carrying the pregnancy to term are not very great.

It would stand to reason, therefore, that the risk of depression is higher among women who experience multiple miscarriages and do not have any other children. With each subsequent loss of pregnancy they see their chances of motherhood slipping away, and as their fear of childlessness increases so too does their risk of experiencing a major depression. But if yearning for a child compounds the risk, ambivalence toward the pregnancy appears to do so as well. In fact, Beutel's study found that depressive symptoms were greater among those women who had been ambivalent toward the pregnancy they lost than they were among those who had wanted and planned it. One can only speculate that the reason for this might be their sense of guilt for having, in effect, gotten what they wished for.

One of the primary risk factors, however, remains a woman's past history of depression. Researchers have found that approximately 54 percent of those who have experienced a past episode of serious depressive illness will relapse after a miscarriage. Not only have I found this to be true among my own patients, but also I find it to be not unexpected in view of the fact that, as we have seen, pregnancy itself frequently triggers the recurrence of depression.

When depression occurs in the wake of a miscarriage, the woman goes through stages of grief that include shock, numbness, preoccupation with the loss, disorganization of thought, and feelings of anxiety. Not surprisingly, she is also often anxious to conceive again. But just as it's important for any woman to wait until her depression is stabilized before becoming pregnant, it's vitally important that any woman who has miscarried address and resolve her feelings surrounding the loss before going on to have another child.

According to one particular report, 86 percent of 221 women who had miscarried became pregnant again within eighteen months, and the majority conceived within six months. For some women, a subsequent pregnancy will help to alleviate grief, but others need to give themselves more time to work through their sorrow in order to prevent the recurrence of depression.

Anna is a midwife of Eastern European extraction who is married to a man who was desperate for a child. When she lost twins at thirteen weeks of gestation, she was naturally upset and sought counseling. Then, while she was still in counseling, she became pregnant again and miscarried at twelve weeks. This time she was shocked, dismayed, and extremely distressed, as well as determined to wait longer before attempting to conceive yet again. Her husband, however, couldn't understand Anna's degree of distress and immediately began to attempt another pregnancy. Again she lost the pregnancy, this time at seventeen weeks. At that point the Recurrent Pregnancy Loss Clinic at the hospital where I work referred Anna to me.

After many counseling sessions with Anna and her husband, I was finally able to make him understand that she was not only dealing with the bereavement associated with pregnancy loss but also experiencing clinical symptoms of depression.

I was delighted, therefore, when I received a call from Anna telling me that she was more than twenty weeks pregnant and would be coming to see me in her third trimester to monitor her medication. Happily, she now has a lovely baby girl who, she says, is a bundle of joy. Anna is content and loving every moment of motherhood!

Even a successful pregnancy following a previous loss can be problematic, however. A study completed by Franche and Mikail in 1999 compared thirty-one pregnant women who had experienced a previous perinatal loss with a control group who had not, and found that those who had miscarried reported higher scores on the Beck Depression Inventory and more depressive symptomology in their next pregnancy. In addition, other studies, including one done by J. A. Hunfield and colleagues in 1997, indicate that those who lose their babies at twenty weeks or later in the pregnancy (perhaps because they have developed a stronger attachment to the fetus) have a greater risk of depression in their following pregnancy than those who miscarried earlier. When this occurs, the mother's mental and emotional state can affect her ability to develop an attachment to the healthy fetus and a stable relationship with the infant.

Kamila, a lawyer, and her husband, a judge, had waited many years to conceive, so when she became pregnant at thirty-eight years of age, it was a momentous occasion. When she lost her pregnancy at close to twenty-four weeks, it was an equally tremendous blow. Not even three months later Kamila was pregnant again. Although this second pregnancy was planned, she started to experience symptoms of severe anxiety that awakened her in the middle of the night. After giving birth to a healthy baby boy her symptoms actually became worse.

Finally, a physician friend of Kamila's husband called and asked me to see her on an emergency basis. The woman who came to my office was anxiety-ridden, deeply sad, and full of shame. She told me that she was experiencing recurrent dreams of her previous pregnancy, and the mental image of her lost baby was keeping her up at night. In fact, Kamila was suffering a postpartum depression so severe that she required hospitalization. Clearly, she should not have become pregnant so soon after her loss because she was not capable, mentally or emotionally, of dealing with her pregnancy.

For a long time she had ambivalent feelings toward her baby and had a difficult time bonding with him. Ultimately, she had to work with a child/infant psychiatrist who is a consultant to our program to help her with attachment and the bonding process. Happily, Kamila's son is now five years old, and despite her busy law practice, she takes him to a parent-participatory kindergarten three times a week.

Even women who do wait, however, can experience complications. And if they have a previous history of depression, they will certainly require close monitoring. Rachel, for example, had suffered two miscarriages and had a history of depression. After her second pregnancy loss she was terrified of experiencing another and was determined to wait two full years before trying again. She took a year's leave of absence from her job, practiced various relaxation techniques, and made sure that she followed a nutritious diet. She was determined that nothing would compromise her third pregnancy.

Some things, however, are simply beyond anyone's control. While she was pregnant, Rachel's husband received a promotion that would require their moving across the country, and because she feared losing the support systems she'd so carefully built, she decided to remain behind and rejoin him after she gave birth. Luckily, she had a strong network of family and friends, because without them she might not have survived the complications that ensued when, in her third trimester, her blood pressure shot up and she had to be hospitalized on complete bed rest. In the hospital her mood was also monitored on a daily basis, and, with close medical supervision, she gave birth to Josh, a healthy baby boy, and joined her husband six months later.

The support of understanding family and friends is essential for anyone who has experienced a loss, but for women who have lost a baby it can have a tremendous impact on their ability to recover. Many of these women find it difficult to socialize or to be in the company of women who are pregnant or have children. They become reclusive, withdrawn, and completely unable to find any joy in their life. They may also find it particularly difficult to deal with people who knew about their pregnancy and are aware of their loss.

Janet was a physician with a busy practice in a small community where virtually everyone knew her. Because of her demanding schedule she wasn't able to take time off from work when, on two occasions, she became pregnant and subsequently miscarried in her first trimester. As a result, many of her patients were aware of both her pregnancies and their loss. Although everyone in the community was supportive and wanted to be there for her, Janet was simply unable to cope with their well-meaning overtures and ultimately took a medical leave of absence and moved to the city, where she could be anonymous and deal with her emotions without feeling that someone was always looking over her shoulder. She is now engaged in intensive counseling and, she hopes, will eventually be able to return to her community and her practice.

What women, their partners, and their health care providers need to understand is that whatever the physical causes or consequences of pregnancy loss, the primary psychological complication is almost always grief, which may turn into depression, which requires professional counseling and, depending on the severity and circumstances, sometimes medication.

Unplanned Pregnancy: The Depression of a Life Disrupted

If the depression of infertility or miscarriage can be seen as a manifestation of loss, the depression that is sometimes attendant upon unplanned pregnancy can be described as the function of a life interrupted or simply derailed.

While researchers have already established that unplanned pregnancy is one of the most important risk factors associated with postpartum psychiatric problems, it is also of serious concern to those of us who are aware of the risk for antenatal depression. Despite the fact that unplanned pregnancies are sometimes associated with women of low economic or educational level, any woman, no matter her situation, can find herself unexpectedly pregnant either because her contraception failed or because she was simply careless.

Fifty or sixty years ago, when contraception was far less reliable, accidental pregnancies were common, and in many cultures women had virtually no say in when or how often they became pregnant. These days, of course, many women aspire to complete their higher education and to have a career outside the home. They expect to plan their pregnancy at a time when it is most convenient and least likely to interfere with other aspects of their lives. When a woman like this becomes pregnant accidentally, it can be a tremendous disruption, and her distress can easily lead to the onset of depression. One might think that having relatively easy access to legal abortion would alleviate rather than exacerbate the problem of what to do in this situation. In reality, however, making that decision can, in and of itself, create the emotional climate that puts a woman at risk—particularly if she and the child's father disagree.

Annie, for example, was in a relationship with a man totally driven to achieve advancement in his career. When I met Annie, her first child was seventeen months old. She told me that the pregnancy was unplanned but that her partner, Dave, had reluctantly gone along with it because he thought it was "the thing to do," and they had planned to be married once the baby was born. Now, however, she had accidentally conceived again, and Dave, who was furious that she'd refused to terminate the pregnancy, had packed his bags and left.

When she came to my office, toddler in tow, she was terrified and cried throughout the entire session. Although she'd initially been hopeful that Dave would return, she hadn't heard a word from him and was now suffering bouts of insomnia and nightmares about her worst fears having come true.

In Annie's case, this second unplanned pregnancy had destroyed her relationship and the family unit she'd hoped to establish with Dave. To see her through the pregnancy, we put her on one of the newer antidepressant medications and monitored her throughout. A year later, she has accepted her situation but is still receiving counseling and continuing to take medication. Although she has put her life back together, it will never be what she had hoped before her unplanned pregnancy knocked it off its track.

Sometimes, of course, going through with an unplanned pregnancy can have a happy outcome, even when the circumstances would seem to predict otherwise. When Laurie, a law student, became pregnant as the result of a one-night stand (even though she was taking oral contraceptives and had also been told she would never conceive because of her chronic endometriosis) she was actually overjoyed. As it turned out, Jackson, the father, was also thrilled, and the two of them decided to get to know each other better as Laurie's pregnancy advanced. But despite the fact that she'd never considered not having the baby and was receiving emotional support from Jackson, Laurie began to experience mood swings and became clinically depressed at the end of her second trimester. She was, however, extremely open to treatment, gave birth to a healthy baby, and now, two years later, is happily married to Jackson.

In both of the cases cited above, the woman decided to go through with her pregnancy, but sometimes the choice is termination. Recently I saw Jade, a professor who had been shocked to learn that she'd conceived at the age of forty-two. She was already the mother of two little girls, ages five and seven, and had suffered postpartum depression after each of those pregnancies. She was stable on antidepressant medication, happy with both her children and her work, and terrified of going through another pregnancy. After evaluating all the pros and cons, she and her husband, who was also a busy professor, made a mutual decision to terminate the pregnancy. A month afterward, when I saw her again in my office, Jade said, "Dr. Misri, the choice I took was a difficult one; I agonized over it for days on end. I can't tell you whether I will regret this later in life, but for now I feel relieved." In this particular case, Jade had carefully considered her options and felt she had made the right decision.

When a pregnancy is unplanned, the expectant mother always has a choice—to go through with the pregnancy or to terminate it. For some women, of course, there will be no choice. There are many who for moral, religious, or other personal reasons simply wouldn't consider termination. But then they are left to cope with this unexpected disruption in their life, and even if they truly want the child they are carrying, the stress of dealing with what will surely be an unforeseen complication can sometimes trigger depression.

Conversely, however, there are also those who know with equal certainty that they can't, for whatever reason, have a child at the time they become pregnant. For them there may also be no choice, but that doesn't mean the decision to terminate their pregnancy is made without much anxiety, sadness, and pain—and that, too, can create a climate in which depression is likely to germinate and grow.

Although both infertility and miscarriage are biological problems, and the decision about whether or not to terminate an unplanned pregnancy is certainly a choice, it is primarily the psychosocial stresses (in combination with a genetic susceptibility) incurred by these situations that cause them to be associated with depression—in much the same way that marital conflict, abuse, and parental loss affect emotional stability. In the following chapter, however, we will be looking at the ways in which actual physical illness can affect or complicate antenatal depression and its treatment.

6

Is It "All in Her Head"?

WHEN THE PHYSICAL
MASKS THE EMOTIONAL

When things go wrong medically in a pregnancy, obstetricians are prepared. They know what to look for and know how to treat it. But for women with emotional problems, that knowledge, in and of itself, can sometimes be as dangerous as the proverbial two-edged sword. The physician may be so concerned with the medical problem that he or she overlooks the accompanying emotional issues—particularly antenatal depression. Or the multiple medical complaints for which the woman seeks help may actually be masking her true problem, which is very often depression.

Historically, women who became mentally ill either during pregnancy or in the postpartum period didn't just go untreated; they might also actually be locked in prisons for the criminally insane. One particularly grotesque example of this occurred when prison doors were flung open in the wake of the French Revolution and many women emerged with their now fully grown children in tow. And according to ancient Anglo-Saxon law, which survived even in the United States until the nineteenth century, women were considered their husbands' property and could be committed to an asylum for committing any act of "disobedience," which might well include symptoms of mental illness (or the husband's perception of such). Although such cruel and unusual punishment is a thing of the past, there remains a dangerous bias among many health care providers who seem, misguidedly, to believe that when a woman is pregnant she suddenly, magically, becomes immune to emotional distress.

Even more problematic is the fact that women themselves—perhaps because they believe they "should" be feeling happy and content—are reluctant to report any other kind of feeling to their health care provider. They don't want to say, "I'm feeling sad," or "I'm feeling anxious," and so they report physical symptoms instead. They might complain of a sore back or an upset stomach or pain in the legs when what they're really trying to say (without saying it) is "Help me! I feel terrible. I'm not enjoying this pregnancy, and I don't know what's wrong with me." Or, conversely, the very fact that they *are* experiencing a variety of uncomfortable or debilitating physical problems will put them at greater risk for depression simply because their physical problems are preventing them from enjoying their pregnancy. The bottom line is that a number of studies indicate a direct association between increased physical complaints and the increased likelihood of emotional problems during pregnancy.

Depression in Disguise

One study conducted in Seattle, Washington, by Dr. Rosemary Kelly and colleagues found an increase in the physical symptoms among pregnant women who were simultaneously diagnosed with psychiatric disorders. In another study, one-third to one-half of the physical complaints reported at a particular outpatient clinic could not be diagnosed as having any medical cause. Dr. Wayne Katon at the University of Washington Medical School in Seattle also found that in an outpatient setting where patients were seen for physical complaints, 80 percent were psychiatrically ill. The most common unexplained medical symptoms reported by these patients were back pain, stomach pain, nausea, headaches, shortness of breath, gastrointestinal problems, leg or joint pain, a pounding heart, dizziness, chest pain, and fainting.

But other research has shown that among medical patients in general, those with six or more physical complaints are three times more likely than those with fewer complaints to be at risk for mood or anxiety disorders. In other words, their physical problems put them at risk for developing psychological or emotional problems. So it would seem that while those who complain of multiple unexplained physical complaints may be suffering some kind of psychiatric illness, a multiplicity of physical problems may also put people at risk for emotional illness.

Given the fact that researchers have been able to document this link between multiple or increased physical complaints and the incidence of depressive illness among pregnant women as well as in the general population, both women and their health care providers need to be aware that any significant increase in medical symptoms may be not a normal response to pregnancy but rather a signal that the woman is having mental or emotional problems.

I recently had the opportunity to give a talk to doctors at a small-town hospital in the interior of British Columbia. Afterward, two busy obstetricians (the only two working in the area) who had taken time from their practices to attend my lecture came up and thanked me for providing them with what they termed "new but hidden" information about antenatal depression. They, too, were frustrated by the fact that their high patient volume sometimes prevented them from taking those few extra minutes to ask the right questions. And, with relation to the overlap of physical and psychological symptoms, one doctor exclaimed, "When we don't know how to distinguish between symptoms of depression and signs of normal pregnancy, it is impossible to determine if our patients are ill or not!" I do appreciate that this can be difficult, because—contrary to the conventional wisdom—it's not just men who find it hard to share their feelings. Many women also have a problem with that, and pregnant women in particular can find it difficult to attach whatever distress they're experiencing to their emotions. As a result, they find it much easier to talk about backaches or stomach problems.

Not so long ago, I worked with a young woman who appeared to be totally and obsessively focused on each and every part of her body. She came to my office every two weeks throughout her entire pregnancy, and each time I carefully documented her complaint of the day. In the end, I had a list of seventy-eight different symptoms, and never once in all that time did this woman say to me "Dr. Misri, I'm depressed. I'm feeling anxious. I'm just not feeling emotionally well." Instead, she took comfort in feeling dizzy or having pains in her legs.

The problem is that many physical symptoms, as we've already discussed, could be either those that normally occur during pregnancy or equally normal symptoms of depression. So when a patient presents these complaints, she may actually be displacing emotional problems she is unable or unwilling to recognize. Alternatively, she may not confess to her true feelings because she is simply too embarrassed by the stigma that is still attached to mental disorders, particularly with relation to pregnancy or mothering. We need to eradicate this stigma once and for all, if for no other reason than that it increases the number of women whose antenatal or postpartum depression goes undiagnosed.

At a women's health conference I attended about a year ago, three brave women who had suffered postpartum depression got up to tell their stories to the audience. Kelly's story, though heartbreaking, is, sad to say, not as unusual as one might think. Kelly came from a small farming community where she had both a large extended family and a great deal of support from friends and neighbors. Yet she perceived herself as completely alone with her depression and described herself as feeling "frozen." All she could do was to repeatedly complain about backaches and headaches to her obstetrician, who in turn kept telling her not to worry. In fact, he had no clue that her repeated presentation of these physical symptoms was the only way she knew or was able to beg for help. When I spoke to her after the meeting she described to me the terrible shame she felt when she was finally diagnosed and hospitalized with a serious postpartum depression, which, in retrospect, she strongly believed had really begun in pregnancy.

Depression is an *illness*, and to think that because it attacks the mind and emotions it is something to be ashamed of or embarrassed about is, to me, not only heartbreaking but also dangerous. We need to bring the prevalence of antenatal depression out of the closet and into the light where it can more easily be seen, not only in order to alleviate unnecessary suffering among thousands of women but also to avoid its hiding behind the physical complaints that so often both mask and mark it.

When Depression Goes Undiagnosed, It Takes a Terrible Toll

Dr. Lislott Andersson and her colleagues at a hospital in Sweden recruited 1,734 patients to fill out the PRIME-MD, a questionnaire given to pregnant women attending obstetrical clinics. The researchers found that the responses given by 14.1 percent of the study's population were indicative of some form of psychiatric disorder, the most prevalent being major depression. In addition, however, they found that those who were suffering from a psychiatric disorder also expressed an unusual fear of delivering their baby.

Women who are anxious, depressed, and not feeling confident about themselves also lack confidence in the process of childbirth. Because they are fearful and think of themselves as failures in general, they are terrified that they will also fail in the delivery of their child. Their anxiety may actually lead to the very consequence they are afraid of, because women who are unable to relax and who do not have a positive image of how the delivery process will proceed are also those most likely to have prolonged and difficult labors.

As a public health nurse, Barbara had counseled hundreds if not thousands of pregnant women through emotional problems and difficult deliveries. When she and her husband decided to have a baby and she became pregnant, she quite naturally began to attend the clinic where she worked. Because she knew all the obstetricians, she felt comfortable confiding in them, and she wanted to practice what she preached to her patients by being open and honest about how and what she was feeling.

Over the course of her pregnancy, however, she found herself becoming more and more withdrawn until she stopped going to her doctor and attending prenatal classes altogether. Luckily, because he knew her so well, Barbara's obstetrician realized that something was very wrong.

Eventually she admitted that she'd stopped attending the classes because she knew she was experiencing symptoms of depression and was embarrassed and ashamed to be "one of them." In other words, even to a professional such as Barbara, who worked every day of her life with women suffering antenatal depression, there were "right" and "wrong" groups of patients. Those in the right group experienced no antenatal problems, sailed through labor and delivery, and were, in her eyes, model patients. Unfortunately, Barbara herself was not what she considered a model patient; she experienced mood swings throughout her pregnancy and was now frightened of the delivery process.

In the end, she had a cesarean section, and only with therapy did she eventually come to understand that she could not deliver vaginally because of her unrealistic fear that she wouldn't be able to go through labor. After repetitive negative thoughts such as "What if my uterus doesn't contract? What if my cervix doesn't dilate?" she had finally convinced herself that it actually would not be safe even to attempt a vaginal delivery.

When Depression Leads to Addiction

Undiagnosed depression can also lead to more serious physical complications for the baby as well as the mother, especially when women try to self-medicate with alcohol or drugs. When I met Nellie, she was twenty-nine weeks pregnant and had been referred to me by her family physician, who sensed there was something wrong that he just couldn't put his finger on. She and her husband, Rob, belonged to a young social set among whom the recreational use of crystal methamphetamine (crystal meth) was considered the amusement of choice for a Saturday night.

She was well dressed, stylish, and elegant, but almost from the moment she sat down in my office she seemed uncomfortable and suspicious of me. When she asked me if I was judging her, I thought the question odd. As it turned out, Nellie had good reason to ask it. Her pregnancy had been unplanned, and although her husband was ecstatic,

Nellie herself was not. For one thing, she simply wasn't happy about the changes taking place in her body. She no longer looked good in her regular clothes, and she thought her maternity clothes were awful. As her pregnancy advanced, things went from bad to worse. She became increasingly depressed, and she thought constantly about crystal meth, which, she said, had always given her a tremendous sense of freedom. Eventually, she began to use it to make herself feel better about her pregnancy.

One day her husband, who had become suspicious of her behavior, arrived home early from work to find her in a state of almost total collapse. Frightened and horrified, he rushed her to the doctor. But even he couldn't bring himself to confide the truth of what was going on and more or less left it up to their family physician to figure things out for himself. That's where I entered the picture.

Somewhat to my surprise, Nellie continued to keep her weekly appointments with the counselor at our hospital who was helping her overcome her addiction while we also began to treat her depression. She and her husband realized that they had narrowly escaped a disaster and could no longer ignore her problem. In the end—much to their relief—Nellie gave birth to a healthy baby girl.

Whatever their drug of choice, be it crystal meth, cocaine, prescription medications, or alcohol, women who self-medicate are not only hurting themselves but also putting the babies they are carrying at risk for complications in utero and at birth. The newborns can develop withdrawal syndromes at birth or develop abnormally, resulting in disorders such as fetal alcohol syndrome. That, of course, is yet another reason why it is so important that we identify and diagnose antenatal depression as early as possible.

Women do not get depressed and abuse drugs or alcohol out of choice or because they are bad people. Rather, when the darkness of depression overtakes them and their judgment is impaired, they don't know how or where to ask for help, and so they do the only thing they know to alleviate their pain. If they don't know what's wrong with them and their doctors don't recognize it, they simply do what they can to escape the reality of depression in whatever way and for however long they can.

If the reporting of multiple physical symptoms is often an indication of underlying depression, and if depression can, in turn, lead to physical complications for mother and child, it's also true that the symptoms of physical illness can both contribute to and complicate the treatment of depression.

Medical, Emotional, or Both?

We've already discussed the fact that depression may sometimes be overlooked because its symptoms so closely mimic those that occur normally during pregnancy. But it's also true that there are medical conditions whose symptoms may mask those of depression as well as others that can contribute to it. The symptoms of autoimmune thyroiditis, or overactive thyroid, for example, include severe anxiety, tension, and fluctuating mood swings, all of which are also symptoms of depression. And although this particular disease is diagnosed postpartum, there is growing evidence to indicate that its onset actually occurs during pregnancy.

Anemia is one of the more common physical problems whose symptoms, including fatigue, listlessness, and a lack of interest in pursuing one's normal activities, are consistent with those of depression. The depression may be masquerading as anemia, or the patient may be both anemic and depressed at the same time, either of which could delay the proper diagnosis. Doctors in general understand that they need to be on the lookout for anemia during pregnancy. As a result, if a patient complains of symptoms that are generally associated with it, the doctor will treat her for anemia, and it may be some time (perhaps not until she fails to show any improvement) until he or she considers there might be another cause for the woman's symptoms and begins to suspect that the patient could be depressed.

Sometimes when a woman is already dealing with the normal stresses of pregnancy, any physical complication can create just enough additional tension and anxiety to trigger depression. In my own practice, I've seen this happen more than once when, for example, a woman is diagnosed with gestational diabetes.

Pregnancy can cause blood sugar levels to rise, particularly if there is a family history of diabetes. Many women can control gestational diabetes with diet and exercise alone, and they are able to deal with the problem quite well, as they know that it will probably resolve itself once their baby is born. Others, however, may require insulin injections and must constantly monitor their blood sugar and insulin levels to ensure that their diabetes is under control. When this happens, health care providers are likely to overlook the fact that their patient may be struggling not only with her diabetes but also with the coexisting emotional stress of having to inject herself on a daily basis throughout her entire pregnancy. The women I've talked to about this tell me they feel somehow "cheated" and are extraordinarily sensitive to the fact that their pregnancy has not gone smoothly.

If the caregiver is focused on treating an obvious and dangerous physical condition, he or she may simply be unable to see the depression that accompanies it.

Jill, a patient I'd previously treated for postpartum depression, actually had to call me herself when she realized that her depression had returned and she felt that no one was listening to her. Jill had been put on complete bed rest when her blood pressure rose to dangerous levels during the third trimester of her pregnancy and her doctor became worried that she was at risk of developing eclampsia. When her symptoms of depression began and she tried to tell people about them, all anyone had to say was that of course it was depressing to have to lie in bed day after day. Jill, however, knew what real depression felt like, and she was terrified of having to go through what she'd experienced after her previous pregnancy, when her depression was so severe that she had to be hospitalized.

On the telephone, I could hear the desperation not only in her words but also in her voice. "Dr. Misri," she cried, "all the doctors are very concerned about my blood pressure, and I can certainly understand that. They want my baby to be healthy, and that's what I want, too. But nobody is concerned about how I'm feeling emotionally, and that's my biggest concern right now. So please, you've got to help me!"

Here was a woman literally crying out for help. She wasn't pretending everything was fine; she wasn't masking her feelings by complaining of back pain or a headache. In fact, she couldn't have been clearer about what she was feeling, and still she couldn't get anyone to pay attention. Because she recognized the symptoms of depression and I had treated her previously, she was able to call me and seek help on her own. Not all women, however, are in such a fortunate position.

Certainly when a woman has a medical problem that could potentially threaten her health or the health of her baby, her doctor must treat that problem as quickly and carefully as possible. But that doesn't mean that her physical health is more important than her emotional well-being. As I hope I've been making clear all along, not only is emotional distress as debilitating and painful as physical distress, but also it can be equally dangerous to both mother and child. Plus, in and of itself it can lead to additional physical issues or complicate those that already exist. For all of these reasons, early detection of any psychiatric condition is, beyond any doubt, as important as the early detection of physical illness.

7

Dealing with the Many Faces
of Depression

As we all know, the more medical problems or conditions we have, the more difficult it becomes to diagnose and treat them, and the same certainly holds true for emotional or psychiatric problems. We've already discussed the fact that in women depression often manifests itself in atypical ways or in conjunction with other, complicating factors. In terms of psychiatric complications, these are most likely to be anxiety disorders, eating disorders, and bipolar disorder. Although each of these is defined by the *DSM-IV-TR* as a discrete illness, anxiety and eating disorders can often appear in conjunction with depression. Particularly during pregnancy, the challenge of treating two or more psychiatric syndromes appearing at the same time can be formidable for a variety of reasons.

The Many Faces of Anxiety

It's only recently that anxiety disorders have been officially recognized, validated, and defined by the psychiatric community. Many patients—and particularly women—suffering anxiety disorders were simply labeled "neurotic." Although Freud can't be credited with coining the term, he is certainly the one most responsible for popularizing it and for stamping so many of his female patients with its stigma. Now, however, we recognize that anxiety itself has many faces—ranging from social anxiety disorder, generalized anxiety disorder, and panic disorder to obsessive-compulsive disorder and post-traumatic stress disorder. We know that approximately 30 percent of women will experience some kind of anxiety disorder in their lifetime. We know that more women than men are likely to experience anxiety in conjunction with depression. And we know that, more than any other type of psychiatric illness, some forms of anxiety disorder are likely to last a lifetime, with alternating periods of remission and relapse.

Certainly, with all the stresses we experience in everyday life, anxiety is something with which most of us are well acquainted and which we've learned to live with—if not on a daily basis, then at least from time to time. Feeling anxious is a function of simply being human. It's normal to feel anxious before taking an important exam, before giving a speech or making a presentation, even before a happy event such as a wedding. In those situations, anxiety can actually work to our benefit by motivating us to study, to prepare, to plan. The same may be said of pregnancy, which is a period of heightened anxiety in any woman's life. No matter how confident they may be, many women are anxious about embarking upon motherhood. They may be fearful that their baby could be born with some kind of physical problem or deformity, or they may simply fear the pain of labor and delivery. Many women, in fact, prepare for their pregnancy by giving up coffee and/or cigarettes, trying to eat more nutritiously, and generally becoming more fit. Both the anxiety and the preparation are normal reactions to pregnancy. Clinical anxiety disorder, however, is something quite different.

Panic Disorder

Panic disorder, which afflicts approximately 5 percent of women, is characterized by episodes of a truly terrifying cluster of psychological as well as physical symptoms that seem to appear out of the blue and that can last anywhere from a few minutes to a few hours. Panic attacks are characterized by the abrupt, intense onset of at least four of the following symptoms, as identified by *DSM-IV-TR*:

DSM-IV-TR DIAGNOSTIC CRITERIA FOR PANIC ATTACK

1. Palpitations
2. Shortness of breath
3. Sweating
4. Trembling or shaking
5. Chest pain
6. Feelings of choking
7. Nausea or abdominal distress
8. Feeling dizzy, light-headed, or faint
9. Feelings of being detached from one's body
10. Fear of losing control or becoming crazy
11. Fear of death
12. Unusual numbness or tingling in various parts of the body
13. Chills or hot flashes

Adapted from the American Psychiatric Association, *Diagnostic and Statistical Manual of Mental Disorders, 4th ed., Text Revision (DSM-IV-TR)* (Washington, D.C.: American Psychiatric Association, 2000).

To complicate matters, these attacks can occur with or without agoraphobia—the fear and avoidance of places where escape or assistance might be difficult or embarrassing. Although the term implies fear of open spaces—from the Greek *agora*, an open market or public square, and *phobia*, an irrational fear—people can actually fear and avoid many spaces, open or not, from bridges and tunnels to airplanes and movie theaters. For those who are agoraphobic, a panic attack might be triggered either by being in the place or situation that is feared or by the anticipation of having to be in such a place or situation.

Without agoraphobia, a panic attack may come on without any obvious stimulus at all. That can be even more frightening, as it was for

Annette, who had never experienced one until she was twenty-eight years old and twelve weeks pregnant. Her husband, Rick, was in Europe on business when she awakened in the middle of the night drenched in sweat with severe heart palpitations, acute shortness of breath, and the feeling that her chest was being crushed. Terrified, she called 911 and was rushed to the nearest emergency room, where she was immediately put on a heart monitor and an extensive cardiac workup was begun. When Rick arrived the next day, having caught the first available flight, he found his fit and presumably healthy wife hooked up to machines, undergoing scans, ultrasounds, and other sophisticated tests, and now thoroughly convinced that she had had a heart attack. After two days during which both Annette and Rick were confused and afraid, all the tests proved negative and she was sent home with a clean bill of health.

Needless to say, they both breathed a sigh of relief, but just three weeks later, while Annette was at work preparing a difficult cost analysis for a client and feeling overwhelmed by all the figures in front of her, her vision suddenly blurred, she became dizzy, and she thought she was about to faint. She tried to talk herself out of it by saying, "Annette, get ahold of yourself, you're not going crazy," but she had to leave work and return to her home, a safe place where no one would see how anxious she was. This time she knew she wasn't having a heart attack. Subsequently, she was seen by one of our psychologists, who treated her with cognitive behavior therapy to help her cope with what she now realized were panic attacks.

PANIC ATTACKS DURING PREGNANCY: A CHALLENGE TO DEAL WITH

Like Annette, most pregnant women who experience panic attacks make several trips to the emergency room and are often investigated for heart attacks before being diagnosed with panic disorder. The attacks generally occur just before bedtime, in the middle of the night, or upon awakening, and they are always all-consuming and totally petrifying.

Unlike depression, symptoms of panic do not creep up silently; rather, they arrive like a bolt from the blue and cannot be overlooked or ignored. When I speak to the partners of patients who have panic attacks, they are likely to describe what they've witnessed as something like this: "Angela was in the kitchen peeling vegetables. One minute she was happy as a lark, humming to herself, and the next minute she was shaking all over. He face turned red and her pupils dilated until they were huge. She was bending over, holding her chest, and I just thought, 'Oh my God, it's another panic attack.' "

As with depression, earlier studies seemed to indicate that pregnancy somehow protected against panic attacks. In 1987 D. T. George and colleagues reported in the *American Journal of Psychiatry* that a certain number of patients who suffered from panic disorder had improved during pregnancy only to relapse in the postpartum period. The authors' explanation for this phenomenon was that the pregnancy somehow prevented the fluctuation of neurotransmitters that were responsible for the attacks and/or that elevated progesterone as well as some of its breakdown products possessed barbiturate-like properties that had an anti-anxiety effect. In addition, they speculated that pregnancy gave women greater self-esteem and therefore left them less psychologically vulnerable to anxiety attacks. Sadly, however, all these beliefs have proved to be as wrong as the assumptions about pregnancy's protection against depression.

In fact, in one recent study conducted by L. Andersson and colleagues, 1,795 pregnant Swedish women with no prior psychiatric history were screened for psychiatric disorders while attending a routine ultrasound procedure. The rate of anxiety disorder among these women was found to be 6.6 percent, which is significantly higher than the 2 to 4 percent one would expect to find in the nonpregnant population.

Even without the published data, however, it has long been clear to me that the women I was seeing in my practice did not experience relief from panic attacks during pregnancy. If anything, some remained the same while others grew worse—but only a very few of them became better. My observation has been validated by several studies of women who had been diagnosed with panic disorder prior to becoming pregnant and whose attacks either continued or worsened during pregnancy.

In addition, it is generally accepted that those who experience panic attacks during pregnancy are also at increased risk of having symptoms postpartum.

Panic or Depression: Which Comes First?

Many women who experience repeated panic attacks subsequently become depressed, while others may first become depressed and then see their depression complicated by the onset of panic disorder. In either situation, the management and treatment of these women becomes even more challenging than the treatment of either condition alone—especially when the woman is pregnant.

To begin with, we know that anywhere from 19 to 37 percent of those who are depressed never seek treatment of any kind, so it stands to reason that getting a depressed *anxious* person into treatment would be an even greater challenge—a challenge that is made even more difficult when the potential patient is a pregnant woman. Sometimes the difficulty lies with the patient. Many pregnant women, however panicky and anxious they may be, remain reluctant to engage in treatment in the first place or, if they do, to comply over a period of time. And when panic disorder occurs in conjunction with depression, the treatment process becomes longer and more complicated.

But sometimes it is the physician who fails to recognize the woman's symptoms for what they are, or who is reluctant to prescribe medication, if necessary, to a woman who is pregnant. It is not unusual, in fact, for a patient to arrive in my office for the first time frustrated and upset because she believes her obstetrician didn't hear what she was saying or didn't know quite what to do with her. And sometimes the doctor and patient are equally baffled by what she's experiencing, which is just what happened to Serena.

Serena had been diagnosed with hyperthyroidism (an overactive thyroid) several years before, but with medication her disease was under control. Then, despite using contraception, she became pregnant. Serena began to freak out and refused to accept that she had indeed conceived. Many of the symptoms of her thyroid disease, such as fatigue, insomnia, heart palpitations, and increased sweating, began to recur, and because she kept insisting to her doctor that she couldn't possibly be pregnant, they retested her thyroid and also administered a second pregnancy test. The doctor wanted to be certain he hadn't missed diagnosing a medical condition, and in any case it had never occurred to either one of them that Serena might be suffering from panic attacks.

It wasn't until the thyroid tests came back negative and the second pregnancy test was again positive that Serena began to accept not only that she was pregnant but also that the symptoms she was experiencing were related to her pregnancy, not to her thyroid. By this time Serena was ten weeks pregnant and had started experiencing pervasive feelings of sadness together with symptoms of anxiety, which made the diagnosis clearer to her doctor. In fact, it would be quite unusual for a physician to diagnose the onset of pregnancy-related panic attacks and/or depression without first ruling out the possibility of an underlying medical condition, which means, for the pregnant woman, that finding the answer to her problem might take several prenatal visits. Sometimes it can take even longer.

Dorothy, a Native American, was admitted to the hospital because of uncontrollable high blood pressure during her pregnancy. She was in the hospital for more than a week without ever disclosing to any of her caregivers that she'd been having eight to ten panic attacks every single day. In fact, she hid her symptoms very well until a nurse went to check on her one night and found Dorothy sitting up in bed meditating.

When the nurse asked her what was wrong, Dorothy finally broke down and confessed that she was constantly experiencing breathlessness, tingling, and numbness in various parts of her body and that she was afraid she was dying. Luckily the nurse had attended a lecture on anxiety disorders just the week before and so could recognize Dorothy's symptoms for what they really were.

When I saw her the following day, I started her on a low dose of antidepressant medication in addition to the blood pressure medications she was already taking and to which she had not responded. Dorothy remained in the hospital for another three weeks, after which she was discharged with her panic attacks substantially diminished. She has since given birth to a healthy baby and, having waited two years, is now planning a second pregnancy.

In Dorothy's case, the high blood pressure and panic attacks occurred as two separate problems, and the connection between the two still remains unclear. In my psychiatric practice, however, I very frequently see them occur in conjunction with one another, and once the panic attacks are treated, the blood pressure often returns to normal. Dorothy has stopped drinking coffee, exercises regularly, and continues to take her medication. Because she is now aware of her conditions, she will be able to monitor herself carefully during her next pregnancy.

When Anxiety Goes Untreated, the Consequences Can Be Devastating

My hope is that if more patients and their caregivers are aware of the frequency with which anxiety disorders can accompany pregnancy, their diagnosis will be made sooner, thereby reducing the woman's emotional distress and preventing further complications for both mother and child not only during pregnancy but also after birth.

In England, Dr. J. Heron and colleagues completed the Avon Longitudinal Study of Parents and Children in which 8,323 women were twice given the same questionnaire regarding self-reported symptoms of anxiety and depression, once at eighteen weeks of gestation and again at thirty-two weeks. What the researchers learned is that antenatal anxiety is a frequent occurrence, that it often overlaps with symptoms of depression, and that it also increases the likelihood of postpartum depression. Failure to diagnose or to treat the anxiety, therefore, poses a significant risk to both the mother and her baby.

Theresa's story illustrates just how serious that dual risk can be. Theresa had a history of panic attacks and had been taking antidepressant medication to control her illness. When she became pregnant, however, she immediately stopped taking her medication because she erroneously believed—as so many people do—that her pregnancy would protect her from the anxiety. For the first two or three weeks she did feel better. But at about nine weeks she began to feel that her baby was somehow deformed, and the panic attacks returned. Still, Theresa refused to go back on her meds. She was going to yoga classes, taking long walks, and using relaxation techniques, and although her symptoms continued throughout her pregnancy, she was able to control them well enough to make her life reasonably livable.

When her son was born, however, things went from bad to worse. Theresa had a difficult time breast-feeding and was self-conscious because friends kept questioning her about her inability to nurse. Every time she looked at her baby she began to feel anxious, to the point where she could barely bring herself to touch the infant or to establish any kind of positive feeling toward him. Because she felt that the baby himself had triggered her panic attacks in utero, and because she'd visualized him as being deformed, once the child was actually born she couldn't shake the anxiety toward him that had become so firmly entrenched. In the end, she needed treatment with a psychologist who specialized in cognitive behavior therapy in order to be able to love her son without being panicked by him.

Even before her baby was born, however, Theresa may well have been putting him as well as herself at risk by allowing her anxiety to go untreated. Many studies have shown that increased anxiety during pregnancy is often associated with conditions including preeclampsia, preterm labor, and even miscarriage, as well as changes in fetal blood circulation and behavior—all of which I'll be discussing in detail in Chapter 11.

WHEN A CHILD IS TRULY AT RISK

Theresa's baby, thankfully, was born perfectly healthy despite her unfounded fears and untreated anxiety, but sometimes the baby's health truly is compromised, and that, too, can trigger panic in the mother. If you know your baby has a serious medical condition, it would seem only normal to be anxious. At times, however, anxiety can cross the bounds of normalcy into a clinical psychiatric condition, and because of all the sophisticated prenatal testing we are able to do today, any chromosomal abnormality in the baby is diagnosed during pregnancy.

One eighteen-year-old mother was referred to me by her pediatrician because of the uncontrollable panic attacks she'd been experiencing ever since her child was diagnosed with a severe lung disorder in the third trimester of her pregnancy. After she gave birth, as her child underwent a series of medical workups, her panic increased and she became more and more certain he would die. She began to experience severe night sweats and chest pains, and she slept in the baby's room night after night, convinced that he wouldn't survive.

In another, similar case, a mother was told at twenty-one weeks of gestation that her baby had a serious kidney disease, and even though she had no previous history of anxiety, she began to experience breathlessness and the sensation that she was actually choking.

Although it appears reasonable to assume a direct cause-and-effect relationship between the baby's diagnosis and the mother's acute anxiety, we can't at this point prove that these women's panic attacks were caused by their children's illness. Still, it would be safe to suggest that doctors ought to be alert to the possibility that women may suffer severe anxiety when their babies are at serious risk.

Ghosts in the Nursery

When your baby's life is in danger, the fear—whether or not it is accompanied by clinical anxiety—is very much in the present, but experiences in the past, or even long forgotten, can also lead to panic during pregnancy. This syndrome was first described as "ghosts in the nursery" by Dr. S. Fraiberg in 1975 and refers to adverse childhood experiences that have not been explored or resolved and which may therefore trigger severe anxiety with relation to impending motherhood.

While ghosts in the nursery may be a unique variation on panic disorder, other symptoms, such as those Theresa experienced when she feared her unborn child would be deformed, are not unlike the intrusive thoughts that plague women with another form of anxiety disorder—obsessive-compulsive disorder.

Obsessive-Compulsive Disorder

Obsessive-compulsive disorder (OCD) is a psychiatric illness that affects 2 to 3 percent of the general population, with symptoms sometimes beginning as early as age eight. The "obsessive" component of the disorder refers to the person's experience of recurrent, unwanted, intrusive, negative thoughts that produce an enormous amount of distress. The person *knows* these thoughts are not normal yet has no control over them despite all efforts to resist. The obsessions can take on many themes, including concerns about or fear of contamination, aggression or violence, symmetry, sex, religion, and death or illness.

Because these thoughts are so disturbing, the person who experiences them engages in ritualistic behaviors designed to avoid the anxiety they produce. Those acts—the "compulsive" component of the disorder, which might include checking, praying, repeating, counting, and hand washing—then become so compelling that they themselves effectively take over the person's life.

Many OCD sufferers are controlling individuals, and, ironically, the more they attempt to control their environment, the more out of control they become, the more ashamed and embarrassed they are, and the more they try to hide their thoughts even from their loved ones.

DSM-IV-TR DIAGNOSTIC CRITERIA FOR OBSESSIVE-COMPULSIVE DISORDER

A. Obsessions are defined by:

1. Recurrent, persistent thoughts, impulses or images, which are intrusive and inappropriate, causing marked anxiety.
2. Thoughts, impulses, or images that are not simply excessive worries about real-life problems.
3. The person attempts to ignore, suppress, or neutralize the thoughts with some other thought or action.
4. The person recognizes obsessional thoughts to be a product of his/her own mind.

Compulsions are defined as:

1. Repetitive behaviors (e.g., hand washing, checking) that the person is driven to perform in response to an obsession.

2. The behaviors or mental acts are aimed at preventing or reducing distress.

B. The person has recognized the obsessions or compulsions to be excessive and unreasonable.

C. Symptoms cause marked distress, are time-consuming, and significantly interfere with functioning.

D. Symptoms are not due to another psychiatric disorder, such as preoccupation with food in an eating disorder.

E. Symptoms are not the result of substance abuse (e.g., drug or medications).

Adapted from the American Psychiatric Association, *Diagnostic and Statistical Manual of Mental Disorders, 4th ed., Text Revision (DSM-IV-TR)* (Washington, D.C.: American Psychiatric Association, 2000).

While one study indicates that approximately 29 percent of OCD sufferers also have symptoms of phobic illness (excessive fears associated with anxiety) and 14.5 percent abuse or are dependent upon controlled substances, depression is the most common psychiatric illness to occur in conjunction with obsessive-compulsive disorder.

PRENATAL AND POSTPARTUM OCD

When Dr. Jonathan Abramowitz and his colleagues at the Mayo Clinic examined the obsessive, intrusive thoughts of three hundred women and their partners with no previous psychiatric diagnosis following the birth of their baby, they found several common themes, including thoughts of suffocation ("Maybe my baby rolled over and died from SIDS"), thoughts of accidents ("I think of the neighbor's dog attacking my baby"), unwanted ideas of or urges toward intentional harm ("Would she be brain-damaged if I threw her out the window?"), thoughts of illness or losing the infant, unacceptable sexual thoughts ("I thought about the baby's genitals"), and finally contaminations.

As the survey results indicate, intrusive, unacceptable thoughts are common even among healthy new parents. These thoughts, however, are generally not intense, they usually happen in passing, and they do not involve accompanying compulsive or ritualistic behaviors. Full-fledged obsessive-compulsive disorder is quite different.

Given the nature of the illness, it shouldn't be surprising that OCD might occur or recur during pregnancy or when a new mother is concerned about the care and health of her infant. In fact, at least one study indicates that OCD does occur in the postpartum period, often along with generalized anxiety disorder or panic disorder. Again, however, its occurrence during pregnancy has been given far less attention.

Josephina and Joseph, who had been married for many years, were good parents to their two older children when Josephina conceived unexpectedly during a trip to Thailand. After her return home, she started to obsess that fumes she had inhaled in Thailand were toxic and adversely affecting the baby she was carrying. As the pregnancy advanced she tried to tell her pediatrician and her family doctor about her fears, but neither of them paid much attention, and when the baby was born healthy her obsessive thoughts went away.

When she became pregnant again a few months later, however, she once more became obsessed with the thought that her baby was damaged, this time by the lead-paint–coated banisters in her home. But this time, even after the baby was born healthy and normal, those thoughts continued in the postpartum period, and eventually Josephina learned to live with them.

When I finally saw her in my office, thirteen weeks pregnant for the fifth time, she was obsessed with thoughts of a variety of toxic substances she was sure were affecting her baby. No matter how hard she tried to stop them, the thoughts simply wouldn't go away.

As appears to be true of many women during pregnancy and postpartum, Josephina didn't engage in compulsive behaviors to deal with her obsession; she was simply preoccupied with repetitive, troublesome, and intrusive thoughts night and day. At the moment, there is some question as to whether pregnancy-related obsessive thinking unaccompanied by compulsions will lead to full-fledged OCD or whether it is a temporary phenomenon that will be resolved with treatment. In Josephina's case, because the postpartum period remained fraught with severe depression along with intrusive thoughts, she was referred to an anxiety disorders clinic, where she required prolonged treatment.

With or without accompanying compulsive behaviors, however, the obsessive thoughts of women during pregnancy or postpartum generally involve the baby. Anxiety-provoking thoughts of actually harming the child are most common and may involve obsessing about stabbing the newborn with a knife, harming the infant while he is sleeping by accidentally shaking, strangling, or choking him, or inadvertently sexually molesting him by touching him inappropriately. Some of my patients tell me that many of these thoughts are accompanied by horrific, frighteningly vivid images of how the baby gets hurt. For example, some visualize mistakenly throwing their child into the microwave or down a flight of steps, or accidentally driving him into oncoming traffic.

If there are compulsive ritualistic behaviors accompanying these unwanted thoughts or obsessions, they might revolve around making sure the baby is clean by repetitively washing his bottles or clothes, or making sure he is safe by engaging in compulsive checking and rechecking behavior that goes well beyond the normal baby-proofing.

Women with preexisting symptoms of OCD often experience a worsening of their symptoms in pregnancy. In a study of eighty-nine patients with OCD done in the United Kingdom by Malcolm Ingram, 25 percent of the women reported that pregnancy was the single most stressful factor for triggering their symptoms. In another survey of 180 OCD patients conducted at Massachusetts General Hospital by Lynn Buttolph and Amy Holland, close to 70 percent of those who responded indicated a worsening of symptoms associated with either pregnancy or childbirth. My own clinical experience certainly supports these statistics.

Maya, for example was a patient of mine who had been seriously afflicted with OCD since the age of fourteen. She became pregnant while being treated with an SSRI in combination with regular visits to a psychologist for cognitive behavior therapy.

Being in a stable, happy marriage and seeing many of her contemporaries and peers becoming pregnant, Maya decided to become pregnant. Luckily, she was wise enough to continue both her medication and her cognitive behavior therapy. One of her obsessions before becoming pregnant had been the thought that she would sexually touch other women. During pregnancy, this obsession turned into "What if I sexually touch my baby?"

As it happened, when she had an amniocentesis she learned that she was carrying a girl. The thought that she might accidentally sexually touch her baby girl persisted throughout the pregnancy, and after she gave birth her therapist had to make home visits and literally stand by her side to help her with the diaper changes until, with several weeks of this exposure therapy, which is frequently used to treat OCD patients, Maya was able to change her daughter's diaper without help.

OCD and Hormonal Fluctuation

In Chapter 3 I discussed what effect the rise in the levels of estrogen and progesterone during pregnancy might have on serotonin transmission, its reuptake, and its receptor-binding capacity—an effect that could also very well trigger the onset or worsening of obsessive-compulsive symptoms.

Similarly, the onset of postpartum OCD has in some women been found to correlate with a fluctuation in levels of oxytocin and prolactin. Women with severe OCD—especially if they have gone untreated— appear to have higher-than-normal levels of oxytocin in their cerebrospinal fluid. In addition, those with more obsessive-compulsive symptoms appear to have lower-than-normal levels of prolactin.

It seems, therefore, that the more we are able to learn about the neurohormonal triggers of obsessive-compulsive disorder during pregnancy and postpartum, the better understanding we may have of the neurobiology or biological component of obsessive-compulsive disorder in general.

When OCD Is Confused with Psychosis

Any woman who experiences symptoms of OCD during pregnancy or in the postpartum period should feel that she can ask her doctor for help. Sadly, however, many women are afraid to do so because they believe that speaking to someone about their obsessive thoughts or fears of harming their baby will lead to their being declared unfit parents, and they will have their children taken away.

Obsessive symptoms are quite specific in that they are repetitive, unwanted thoughts that the person is *aware* are not normal even though she is unable to stop them. These are very different from psychotic symptoms, where the repetitive, unwanted thoughts are actually delusional and the person who is having them *believes* they are real.

I'll be talking about the dangers of postpartum psychosis later in this chapter. For now, however, the point I want to make is that women with OCD almost never harm their children, while those with postpartum psychosis are in very real danger of doing so. But sometimes the distinction between obsessive thoughts and true psychotic thinking is not so easy to distinguish, and in these cases it is generally best to hospitalize the patient in order to minimize the risk that she will harm her baby.

Felicia is one patient who fell into that category. She had met and fallen in love with Nick, a tour guide, while visiting Vancouver from her native Italy, and when she became pregnant they decided to get married right away. Her parents were well-to-do vintners in the Chianti district of Italy, and, living far away in Canada, Felicia both missed her family and felt guilty about depriving her mother of the pleasure of participating in her pregnancy.

Nick suggested that they invite her mother to come to Canada to see Felicia through her pregnancy, but more than wanting to make his wife happy, he was worried because Felicia was constantly obsessing about the baby's not growing properly and repeatedly getting on the scale to see if she'd gained weight. Her mother's arrival, however, did not put an end to Felicia's obsessive thoughts, and once the baby was born she began to obsess about not having enough milk to nourish the infant.

When I finally saw Felicia, I had to admit her to the hospital. Ironically, the baby was, at that point, losing weight. Consumed by her own anxieties, Felicia was not able to care for her properly. In fact, she'd become very afraid of the baby and had started to avoid her as much as possible.

During the two weeks she was hospitalized, Felicia received both antipsychotic and antidepressant medications. Her symptoms resolved themselves, but we were never able to determine whether she was having obsessive thoughts or her thinking had actually become psychotic.

Felicia's case, however, is unusual, and in most instances, as I've said, we needn't worry about women with OCD harming their babies. In fact, one researcher who believes in an evolutionary theory of obsessive-compulsive disorder has put forward the notion that the ritualistic checking and rechecking behavior of many mothers who suffer from OCD may be their way of protecting the child from any harm.

PREVENTING THE POTENTIAL DANGERS OF ANTENATAL AND POSTPARTUM OCD

OCD, either during pregnancy or postpartum, may lead to the mother's avoiding her baby, and when that happens, attachment and bonding issues become critical. But these unfortunate consequences can be avoided if the illness is detected by primary health care providers during the pregnancy. And to those providers I would go even one step further and emphasize that some patients who exhibit symptoms of antenatal or postpartum depression may also be experiencing symptoms of OCD, because patients with OCD do not openly talk about their illness. They are very often afraid, as I've said, that their babies will be taken away, they are usually filled with shame, and they need to feel safe in order to share their feelings.

If you are suffering from obsessive-compulsive disorder, make sure that you talk to your doctor about the illness before becoming pregnant. If you are already pregnant, talk to your doctor about managing your illness both during pregnancy and in the postpartum period, and by all means identify the people in your life who are willing and able to help and support you.

Post-Traumatic Stress Disorder

If fear and embarrassment are two factors contributing to women's reluctance to confide their symptoms of OCD to their doctor, the fear created by a third form of anxiety—post-traumatic stress disorder (PTSD)—can be even more isolating and distressing. Once known as "combat neurosis," PTSD is characterized by the intrusive reexperiencing of a past traumatic event, avoiding close connections with family and friends, emotional numbing, and, finally, chronic hyperarousal.

Intrusive symptoms generally involve terrible nightmares or sudden painful flashbacks that are sometimes so vivid the person actually feels he or she is going through the trauma again. In order not to relive that pain, the person with PTSD becomes emotionally numb, goes about daily life in a dull, mechanical way, becomes more and more isolated, and generally tries to avoid contact with people or situations that are reminders of the trauma. In addition, he or she is hypervigilant, with exaggerated startle responses and symptoms of extreme fear, including an inability to breathe normally, increased heart rate, nausea, sweating, and feelings of panic, all of which mimic the fear created by the actual experience.

Although it is traditionally thought of as an illness of veterans suffering the physiological and psychological consequences of war, PTSD actually affects an estimated 12.3 percent of all women at some time in their lives and generally results from their having been victims of violence. Among those who were molested in childhood, about 27 percent will suffer PTSD, while among those who are raped or victims of physical violence, 80 percent experience this syndrome. At our own clinic, a recent study has shown that approximately 14 percent of the women referred to us with postpartum depression had a history of sexual abuse.

Despite these alarmingly high figures, however, it is rare for a woman with PTSD to voluntarily disclose her condition to her caregiver. Not only is she embarrassed by what's happened to her, but also simply talking about her symptoms with her health care provider can reactivate the feelings she is trying to suppress. In fact, often one clue that a patient might be a victim of post-traumatic stress is her resistance to treatment. Getting a woman to open up and speak freely about rape, molestation, or physical abuse, therefore, requires the careful establishment of a trusting relationship between patient and health care provider.

PTSD and Pregnancy: When Trauma Resurfaces

Since in women PTSD is most often related to some kind of sexual violence or abuse, it stands to reason that when a woman is pregnant the trauma is most likely to come back to haunt her. This is a time when women undergo pelvic exams as well as examinations of other intimate parts of their body that may trigger flashbacks, nightmares, sleeplessness, hypervigilance, and panic attacks without their even being aware that they are unconsciously reliving a deeply buried horror from the past.

When Vanessa came to see me several years ago in just the second month of her pregnancy, she was requesting a psychiatric evaluation in order to have a cesarean section. At the time, C-sections were performed only if necessary for medical or obstetrical reasons, and if a woman wanted to have one for purely psychological reasons, she was forced to go through rigorous and often embarrassing questioning.

Although I knew immediately that Vanessa was struggling emotionally, I didn't at the time know the cause of her struggle. In compliance with hospital policy, I had to refer her to the ethics committee, which ultimately denied her request. Since she'd refused to provide any reason for her wanting a C-section, their decision didn't come as much of a surprise to me. I continued to see Vanessa during her pregnancy, and when she was in her third trimester I received a frantic phone call from her husband, who told me that she had been up every night sweating and trembling, sleepwalking, talking to herself, and sometimes even screaming or crying out. He knew that whatever she had been experiencing, it was deep-seated, intense, and well beyond his capacity to deal with.

It took many sessions before Vanessa trusted me enough to feel safe confiding her long-guarded secret. What she then told me was that she'd been awakening in the night seeing the image of a man wearing green coveralls and a green cap that were similar to the scrubs doctors wear in the operating room. As I continued to gently encourage her to divulge, she further confessed that this green-clad figure was actually her uncle, who had molested her repeatedly when she was a child.

Years after these incidents but also many years before her pregnancy, when Vanessa was having her first pelvic examination, she experienced her first flashback to the molestation, and ever since that time she'd avoided anyone's touching her genitals or doing intrusive examinations, which was why she'd been so desperate to deliver her baby by cesarean section. She further confided that even sexual intimacy with her husband had been traumatic, although she'd never allowed him to know it.

It is not unusual (or surprising) for women with a history of sexual abuse to prefer female health care providers, particularly when they undergo physical examinations. In an innovative study done by Dr. Julia Seng and colleagues at the University of Michigan, women who had identified themselves as victims of childhood abuse were interviewed with the purpose of determining what they perceived to be optimal maternity care so that the doctors could come up with a useful structure for helping health care providers respond in a positive way to their problem. Based on the information they received, the researchers recommended that when obstetricians are dealing with preterm contractions or excessive vomiting in pregnancy, they should consider the possibility that their patient may be suffering from PTSD. They also determined that it was most important for these women to feel safe both psychologically and physically.

Delia, a patient I met when she was admitted to our hospital, is one who, unfortunately, was not able to find that degree of comfort with her physician. Delia had been sexually abused by her stepfather for ten years and, as a result, was terrified of entering a relationship with a man. Instead, she had chosen a female partner with whom she was very happy, and together they had decided to have a baby through artificial insemination. Once Delia had conceived they decided to attend prenatal classes, and Delia went for routine examinations. During one of these exams, conducted by a doctor who reminded her of her stepfather, she experienced her first flashback to the molestation. From that point on, she began to have panic attacks and to avoid going to any more prenatal exams. She was finally admitted to the hospital when her partner became alarmed because Delia had been experiencing severe chest pains and fainting spells.

Often PTSD sufferers seek to numb their pain by using drugs or alcohol. In a study conducted by Paula Moylan at Johns Hopkins University,

123 pregnant opiate- or cocaine-dependent women with or without PTSD were compared to one another in terms of psychosocial functioning. The results indicated that those with PTSD reported greater need for psychiatric treatment, were more likely to have attempted suicide, and had more previous drug treatments than those without. In addition, the PTSD group was more likely to have an additional, concurrent psychiatric problem and a higher rate of substance abuse than the non-PTSD group. In fact, research has shown that between 24 and 58 percent of substance-dependent women seeking drug treatment are also suffering from PTSD.

Dr. Moylan's study is important particularly because it is one of very few that have looked specifically at PTSD in women who are pregnant. Another, conducted by Dr. C. A. Loveland Cook and colleagues, examined 744 pregnant women in five rural counties in Missouri as well as the city of St. Louis. In their sample, PTSD was found to be the third most common psychiatric condition (the most common being major depression and nicotine dependency). Approximately 7 percent were found to have PTSD severe enough to affect their daily life, and—most shockingly—only a small percentage of these had ever spoken to a health care professional about their condition, with no more than 12 percent ever having received treatment.

The message to be taken from these studies is that PTSD is both more prevalent and less treated than many people believe and that health care providers need to be aware that it may be affecting their pregnant patients. Most important is that those who do have this devastating illness receive appropriate treatment so that they can complete their pregnancy with a positive outcome for both mother and child.

CHILDBIRTH AND PTSD: THE TRAUMA OF DELIVERY

Although PTSD normally results from a trauma in the distant past, there is growing evidence that a difficult childbirth experience can, in and of itself, trigger the onset of this illness. In my own practice I have found that women who have experienced a traumatic birth and who become pregnant for a second time often ruminate about their earlier experience and become increasingly distressed as their pregnancy advances. But PTSD can also occur immediately after the trauma, as it did for Pam.

Pam was carrying twins when, in the third trimester of her pregnancy, she developed a serious complication that resulted in the death of one of the babies. After that, Pam became acutely anxious and angry with her doctors. During her first visit with me, it became clear that she blamed the health care system and believed that she hadn't received proper treatment in the hospital. In fact, however, despite the doctors' attempts to save the second twin, there was nothing more they could have done. In effect, the death of one twin had been virtually inevitable if they were to save the other.

It took many months of intensive psychotherapy before Pam was finally able to accept the truth, which was that she had actually received appropriate and proper obstetrical intervention.

When a woman is so focused on her pregnancy going as planned, as Pam was on having twins, it can be difficult for her to come to terms with any deviation from that plan. An Australian study looked at 499 women at four to six weeks postpartum in order to determine how they perceived the care they had received during childbirth. Thirty-three percent were found to have at least three symptoms of delivery-related trauma, and 5.6 percent met the DSM-IV-TR criteria for PTSD. The researchers concluded that the perception of inadequate care during pregnancy as well as high levels of obstetrical intervention during childbirth were associated with the development of acute trauma symptoms. In addition, they noted that caregivers who deliver babies need to be aware that this can be a serious psychological complication of intrusive birth such as a forceps delivery or a C-section.

Riva, for example, had been determined to give birth at home and had hired a midwife to oversee the delivery. Unfortunately, however, when the baby was found to be in fetal distress, Riva was immediately moved to the local hospital. Even then, Riva continued to resist all obstetrical intervention and remained absolutely determined to have a vaginal birth. In light of her vehement feelings, the obstetricians waited as long as they could without endangering the baby, but ultimately they had to perform a cesarean section. Riva, despite giving birth to a healthy eight-pound baby, was horrified and almost immediately developed symptoms of acute PTSD.

Obstetrical Complications and PTSD

Obviously, no doctor would want any woman to experience unnecessary obstetrical intervention during childbirth, but sometimes such procedures are necessary. Perhaps even more worrisome, however, is the evidence that PTSD may actually be associated with an increased risk of obstetrical complications. After studying 2,219 women of childbearing age, Dr. Julia S. Seng, Ph.D., C.N.M., R.N and her colleagues at the University of Michigan School of Nursing, Ann Arbor, Michigan, found that those with a prior history of PTSD were at risk for developing ectopic pregnancy, spontaneous abortion, excessive vomiting, preterm labor, and compromised fetal growth.

It appears, therefore, that—as with any form of untreated depression or anxiety—the baby as well as the mother is at risk. All the more reason, then, for health care providers to be vigilant in looking for symptoms of PTSD in their patients, and for women to be forthcoming with their physicians about any history of molestation, abuse, or violence, as well as any symptoms they may be experiencing or have experienced in the past.

Eating Disorders

Eating disorders are nearly always marked by an almost fanatical degree of secretiveness. Luckily, however, it appears that more women—especially those who have struggled successfully to conquer their illness—are now willing to speak about the problem in public. Many of us, for example, are aware of the late Princess Diana's bingeing and purging, which became worse during pregnancy, and which also appears to have been associated with postpartum depression.

Bingeing and purging, technically bulimia nervosa, which affects 0.8 to 2.3 percent of women, is the most common of the three major eating disorders. Anorexia nervosa is experienced by 0.2 to 0.7 percent of young women and is characterized by an extreme restriction of food consumption, to the point where the sufferer can appear skeletal. The clinical diagnosis of anorexia, in fact, depends upon the patient's having lost more than 15 percent of her (or far less often his) body weight.

Both bulimia and anorexia appear to be associated with the sufferer's need to establish a degree of control in her life. Because she believes that other aspects of her life are out of control, she seeks to find it in the one place she can, by controlling her food intake and body weight—except, of course, that this is a false sense of control, since in actuality she has virtually no control over the disease itself.

It has been estimated that approximately 5 percent of adolescent and adult women suffer from some kind of eating disorder, and among college students that number rises to 10 percent. If left untreated, anorexia can lead to severe nutritional deficiency, insomnia, loss of bone density, mood changes, fatigue, and even ultimately death as the body's systems begin to break down from lack of nourishment. Anorexia can also negatively impact upon fertility. Bulimia, while not characterized by the same degree of emaciation as anorexia, is associated with serious dental, throat, and intestinal problems, including damage to the esophagus, lungs, and stomach, as well as kidney and heart complications.

The third type of eating disorder, known simply as "eating disorder not otherwise specified," involves periodic bingeing without compensatory purging and is both less prevalent and less dangerous than either bulimia or anorexia.

Certainly, in a society where thinness is revered, where women's sense of self-worth is so often dependent on their being acceptably thin, and where up to 85 percent of all women have dieted at some point in their lives, it shouldn't be surprising that eating disorders are prevalent. In fact, for many women, the ability to control their weight is equated with positive qualities such as determination, discipline, and success.

While some studies have shown a genetic propensity toward eating disorders, there is also, perhaps more significantly, a personality type that appears to make some women more prone than others to this type of illness. They tend to be obsessively perfectionist but also impulsive. They may also be substance abusers and engage in other risk-taking behaviors, including shoplifting and/or promiscuity. Interestingly, there are many professions—dancing and gymnastics, to name just two—that encourage perfectionism as well as thinness. In the perpetual quest to determine which came first, the chicken or the egg, it's interesting to speculate whether women with tendencies toward eating disorders are also drawn to these professions, or whether the demands of the profession create a tendency toward the development of eating problems.

That said, however, what concerns us here is how eating disorders may affect the outcome of pregnancy and, conversely, how pregnancy may affect the course of the disorder.

Pregnancy and Eating Disorders: A Dangerous Combination

For many years we believed that, because they often stopped menstruating as a result of their extreme weight loss, women with anorexia could not conceive. Today, however, we know that some women do ovulate, both while they are actively suffering from the disease and when they are in remission. A study my colleagues and I conducted at our own hospital has shown that many women who are diagnosed with major depression during pregnancy also have an eating disorder.

Dr. David Herzog and his colleagues at the Harvard Eating Disorders Program have been following a group of 246 women with eating disorders for more than twelve years. The results to date indicate that those with an active illness are at greater risk for both cesarean section and postpartum depression, but the researchers have also found that the majority of women in their study had normal pregnancies and gave birth to healthy babies.

Other studies, however, have shown quite different results. One, completed in Toronto by Dr. Donna Stewart, found that women who were symptomatic at conception continued to become worse both during pregnancy and postpartum. In another, during which Dr. M. Brinch and colleagues in Denmark followed fifty anorexic women, the prevalence of premature birth was found to be increased and the incidence of perinatal mortality was six times greater than that of the general population. And finally, Dr. James E. Mitchell and colleagues in Minneapolis who studied twenty bulimic women found that their risk of fetal loss due to miscarriage or neonatal death was considerably higher than that of healthy women.

One question of particular importance is whether pregnancy is likely to improve or worsen an existing eating disorder, and the answer to that seems to be that it can go either way.

Melissa is one for whom pregnancy was associated with relapse. She had begun to suffer from anorexia at the age of fourteen, but she was admitted to a treatment center and was eventually able to control her disease. In fact, having qualified as a nurse counselor in private practice and earning a second degree in nutrition, she herself became a specialist in treating patients with complex eating disorders.

When she became pregnant, however, Melissa began to avoid weighing herself at her prenatal classes. When she occasionally did weigh herself, she either avoided looking at the number on the scale or stood on it backward. When a nurse brought this behavior to the attention of Melissa's obstetrician, he began to monitor her more closely until, in her second trimester, her lack of weight gain prompted him to ask her point blank if she had been restricting her food intake.

At that point, Melissa became quite agitated and refused to pay any more prenatal visits to that particular doctor's office. Luckily, the nurse who had first noticed her peculiar weighing behavior had a sister who'd also been a victim of anorexia, so she knew what devastation it could cause and took it upon herself to make a visit to Melissa's home. With the nurse's encouragement and at her husband's insistence, Melissa went back into treatment and was able to begin eating normally again, gain weight appropriately, and give birth to a healthy baby, although she must still be monitored to be sure she doesn't relapse postpartum.

Postpartum relapse is always a concern, even for women who manage to control their eating disorder during pregnancy. Ruth, for example, appeared to have it all under control. An internationally known watercolor artist, she had grown up in a household where achievement was both expected and revered. Her mother expected perfect order and cleanliness and often criticized Ruth for not cleaning up her room, even though, as Ruth later told me, it was so clean you could "eat off the windowsill." Her father was a world-renowned dentist whose innovative techniques had been cited in textbooks.

Although Ruth, too, excelled in her chosen field, the pressures of growing up in such a competitive environment had led her to deal with her anxieties by bingeing and purging. Her husband, who was relaxed and easygoing—exactly the opposite of what she had grown up to expect from her parents—had no idea what Ruth was doing. He never knew that after he went to bed at night she would eat boxes of cookies and then immediately make herself throw up so that by the next morning she could almost believe it had never happened. Her binges went from cookies to french fries to other junk foods until, just before she became pregnant, she was actually getting in the car after her husband was asleep to buy bags of chips or cookies. She'd then return home with her haul, eat everything she'd bought, throw it all up, put out the garbage, and pretend the next day that she was perfectly fine.

When Ruth became pregnant, however, her bingeing stopped. She felt extremely protective of the baby she was carrying, and throughout her first trimester she remained fully in control of her eating patterns. In her second trimester, the healthy baby she saw on the ultrasound reinforced her determination to look after herself and her child.

After she gave birth, however, everything changed. Ruth became extremely anxious and depressed, and her bulimia returned with a vengeance. With the help of a nutritionist, medications, and group therapy, she was eventually able to control both her depression and her bulimia, but she and her husband have decided not to risk any more pregnancies because the problems she suffered postpartum were so devastating to her and her family.

Obviously, if a woman does not receive adequate nutrition during pregnancy, or if she is constantly purging, her behavior can have disastrous consequences for her baby. But another serious concern we have as medical professionals is that women who severely restrict their own eating might also become restrictive of their babies.

In one such case, the public health nurse who was making a postpartum home visit (a practice that is routine in both Canada and Australia) noticed that her patient, Trisha, was giving the baby her breast for no more than a minute before announcing, "Now I'm done." After monitoring the situation for a period of time, the nurse found that the baby was rapidly losing weight. At that point she became quite concerned and called the family doctor, who referred Trisha to me.

As I learned during our sessions together, Trisha had wanted to be sure that her baby, Angelica, was adequately fed, but she was equally concerned that she not become fat. Trisha described herself to me as having been a chubby child who was constantly teased during elementary school. When she reached puberty she had learned to control her weight through vigorous exercise and extremely restricted eating. She joined the track team and was so good that she later competed internationally and, through her running, managed to shed two stigmas at once: her excess weight and the lack of respect she believed she'd received from her peers.

Her pregnancy had been perfectly planned, the delivery went perfectly, and her baby was the perfect weight. And yet she continued to have visions of Angelica's turning into a "fat little Trisha." The only way she could see to prevent this from happening was by making sure that the baby didn't feel too hungry at the outset, as she recalled she had done as a child, and as her mother had kept reminding her by telling her how much she'd eaten as a baby. What she simply didn't realize was that by restricting Angelica's food intake she was actually jeopardizing her health. Trisha, based on her own past experience and feelings about herself, actually thought she was doing the right thing.

With medication, psychotherapy, and working with an eating disorders specialist, Trisha was ultimately able to control her own eating behaviors and to understand the risk at which she'd been putting her own baby, but her story illustrates the lack of control, as well as the frustration and depression, associated with eating disorders, not to mention the physical risk the eating problems themselves can create for both mother and child.

As with any emotional or psychological problem, particularly when a woman becomes pregnant, the sooner her health care provider is aware of it, and therefore of the possible complications it might create, the less likely it is that the health and safety of both mother and child will be compromised. Therefore, any woman who has a history of an eating disorder—even if she believes it is all in the past—needs to share that information with her doctor. And physicians need to be aware of potential warning signs, which might be any strange or unusual reaction to routine weighing, any sign that the fetus is not gaining weight as it should be, any history of infertility or lack of menstruation, a previous unexplained spontaneous pregnancy loss or neonatal difficulty, unusual or uncontrollable vomiting, or any history of physical or sexual abuse, which is often associated with a subsequent eating disorder.

As I've said and will continue to emphasize, when it comes to ensuring a healthy and safe pregnancy, with a positive outcome for both mother and child, being aware of a woman's psychiatric history is as important as knowing any other aspect of her medical history. Unrecognized and untreated depression—whether or not it is accompanied by the complications of anxiety disorder, post-traumatic stress disorder, or an eating disorder—can compromise that positive outcome as surely as any undiagnosed physical condition. And that is particularly true when the woman is suffering from bipolar disorder, which is characterized by severe mood swings that, if untreated, can lead to psychosis and the kinds of postpartum tragedies that have become all-too-familiar newspaper headlines in the last several years.

The Risks of Bipolar Disorder

Approximately two million American adults, about 1 percent of the population age eighteen or older, suffer from bipolar disorder every year. Unlike depression unaccompanied by mania, bipolar disorder seems to strike women later than men. Like depression, however, it appears to be triggered by a number of factors, including family history, personality type, environmental factors (such as degree of psychosocial support), stressors such as childbirth, and the hormonal changes women experience during their childbearing years.

Also known as "manic-depressive illness," bipolar disorder encompasses a range of moods that are best expressed as a continuum.

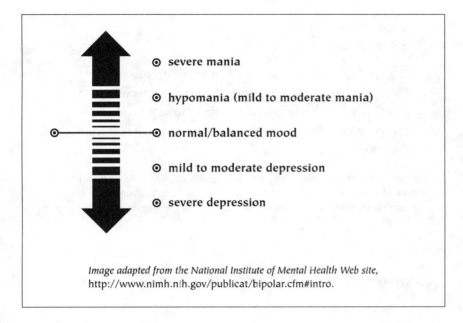

Image adapted from the National Institute of Mental Health Web site,
http://www.nimh.nih.gov/publicat/bipolar.cfm#intro.

As is true of virtually all psychiatric disorders, diagnosing bipolar disorder is a matter of recognizing the point at which the normal ups and downs we feel from day to day step over the line, so to speak, into clinical illness.

The following describes the *DSM-IV-TR* diagnostic criteria for mania:

DSM-IV-TR DIAGNOSTIC CRITERIA FOR MANIC EPISODE

A. A period lasting at least one week of abnormally and persistently elevated, expansive, or irritable mood.
B. At least three of the following symptoms must be present:

1. Increased energy
2. Restlessness
3. Excessive high feeling, unusually happy, or euphoria
4. Extreme irritability
5. Racing thoughts, speediness, talking very fast
6. Little sleep

7. Unrealistic beliefs
8. Poor judgment

C. The symptoms don't also include a mixed episode.
D. The symptoms cause impairment in social or occupational functioning; may intend to cause harm to self or others.
E. The symptoms are not due to substance use or a medical condition.

Adapted from the American Psychiatric Association, *Diagnostic and Statistical Manual of Mental Disorders, 4th ed., Text Revision (DSM-IV-TR)* (Washington, D.C.: American Psychiatric Association, 2000).

Conversely, the criteria for clinical depression are as follows:

DSM-IV-TR DIAGNOSTIC CRITERIA FOR MAJOR DEPRESSIVE EPISODE

A. Five or more of the following symptoms experienced most of the day, nearly every day, for two weeks or more:

1. Feeling sad, empty, and helpless
2. Extreme feelings of guilt, worthlessness, and hopelessness
3. Loss of interest and pleasure in activities once enjoyed, including sex
4. Decreased energy, feelings of fatigue
5. Sleeping too much, change of appetite
6. Restlessness and irritability
7. Difficulty concentrating, remembering
8. Chronic pain
9. Thoughts of death or suicide

B. The symptoms don't also include a mixed episode.
C. The symptoms cause significant distress or impairment in social and/or occupational functioning.
D. The symptoms are not due to substance use or a medical condition.

E. The symptoms are not caused by the loss of a loved one, and persist for two months.

Adapted from the American Psychiatric Association, *Diagnostic and Statistical Manual of Mental Disorders*, 4th ed., *Text Revision (DSM-IV-TR)* (Washington, D.C.: American Psychiatric Association, 2000).

In today's society, terms such as *psychotic* and *manic* tend to be bandied about loosely, along with *wacko* and *crazy*, but *psychosis* and *mania* are clinical terms with specific meanings that denote particular conditions, and it makes me upset to hear them used casually as pejoratives in cocktail party conversation. *Psychosis* denotes a state of unreality along with perceptual disturbances of hallucinations such as hearing voices or seeing or sensing the presence of things not actually there. It also includes delusions, strongly held false beliefs, and other illogical thoughts. It may accompany hypomania (a mood state in which the person is not frankly manic but is experiencing manic symptoms in a somewhat milder form), mania, or depression.

To complicate bipolar disorder even further, people may experience a mixed episode, which involves both manic and depressive symptoms being expressed simultaneously. A woman, for example, might feel sad and hopeless but at the same time extremely energized. This mixed state is of particular concern for women of childbearing age because it is often accompanied by psychosis and suicidal thinking. When I see a woman whose thinking and behavior have changed so drastically, that is the one time I never hesitate to hospitalize a patient—for her own safety as well as that of her child.

In addition, the illness manifests in a variety of forms. Classic bipolar disorder is characterized by recurrent episodes of mania and depression with periods of normalcy in between. In another form, there are periods of milder hypomania alternating with depression. In rapid-cycling bipolar illness, which generally develops later in the course of the illness and more frequently in women than in men, four or more episodes of either mania or depression occur within a single twelve-month period.

Bipolar Disorder, Pregnancy, and Postpartum Psychosis

Recently Marlene Freeman and colleagues in Tucson, Arizona, looked at the way reproductive events impacted the course of bipolar disorder in women and found that of the thirty study participants who had given birth, twenty experienced a postpartum psychotic episode. All of those who had such an episode after the birth of their first child also had one after the birth of subsequent children. The researchers concluded that hormonal fluctuations were associated with an increased risk of episodic fluctuation of mood in women with bipolar disorder.

In fact, women with bipolar illness are at high risk for relapsing in the postpartum period, are seven times more likely than the general population to require hospitalization for their first episode of post-partum depression, and have a hundredfold higher risk for developing postpartum psychosis.

As far back as 1838 Jean Etienne Dominique Esquirol was documenting cases of mental illness in childbearing women in France, and in 1858 another French physician, Louis-Victor Marcé, published *Traité de la Folie des Femmes Enceintes*, a treatise on emotional disorders during pregnancy and after delivery. So it seems that for more than 150 years doctors have been aware of and puzzled by this baffling phenomenon.

Postpartum psychosis occurs suddenly in one to two of every one thousand women after childbirth and is now believed to be closely linked to—if not actually a variant of—bipolar illness. In a review of sixteen studies on postpartum psychosis Dr. Emma Robertson found that anywhere between 39 and 81 percent of women who experienced their first psychotic episode postpartum continued to experience subsequent episodes that were not linked to childbirth. A longitudinal follow-up study by the same researcher reported that 86 percent of 110 women diagnosed with a postpartum psychotic episode subsequently met the criteria for bipolar disorder. As a result, she concluded, as have others, that post-partum psychosis is not a discrete illness but rather a post-partum presentation of an underlying mood disorder. My own findings in my practice are that once a woman has experienced an episode of postpartum psychosis, the eventual course of her illness is no different from the classic form of bipolar disease.

Researchers are now looking for a potential genetic link between bipolar disorder and postpartum psychosis because those who have a family history of psychosis develop the disease at twice the rate of women who don't.

The danger, of course, is that when postpartum psychosis does occur, both mother and child are at serious risk. It appears virtually out of the blue, with acute instability of mood, often hypomania, disorganized behavior, and—most seriously—hallucinations and/or delusions, usually revolving around the infant. These women are often preoccupied with thoughts of harming their baby, and many of them are, in fact, in danger of acting out their thoughts. Because of that, physicians need to understand that when a woman is depressed in the postpartum period, and particularly if her depression has a psychotic component, it is always a medical emergency. In bipolar women, the depression can switch to mania so quickly that very often even the woman's partner doesn't have time to see it coming—which is exactly what happened in Tina's case.

Tina is an occupational therapist who works with mothers and children on a daily basis. Her husband, Robert, is a college professor, and they have a very good, stable marriage. When they determined the time was just right, Tina became pregnant.

Robert, however, had recently been promoted, was extremely busy with his students, and was likely to be interrupted by one of them, even at home, at any hour of the day or night. Tina therefore decided that once her baby was born, she would go to live with her mother for a while in order to have the uninterrupted help and support she would need at that time. Her mother had prepared a bedroom for her and had even hired a nanny. What Tina didn't know, however, because it had never been discussed, even among family members, was that her mother had suffered an acute episode of postpartum psychosis that had required hospitalization, and she was very much aware that Tina was at risk for developing the same illness.

Sure enough, during the third week of her stay, Tina began to develop what her mother immediately recognized as signs of postpartum psychosis. She was unusually happy, to the point of seeming euphoric, and was going on shopping sprees virtually every day, buying huge quantities of outfits the baby didn't need. By the end of the episode, she'd accumulated more than five hundred pieces of infant clothing.

The escalation of her mood occurred so rapidly that by the third day she started to become irritable and hostile, vehemently denying there was anything wrong. Because she was unable to sleep, she stayed up all night making grandiose plans for herself and the baby. At that point, both her husband and her mother knew that she had to be hospitalized. She was admitted immediately, and I personally oversaw her care, treating her and administering the medications, lithium in particular, that stabilized her mood. She was discharged feeling completely well, and I continued to monitor her condition for more than a year.

Both women and their physicians need to understand how important that follow-up monitoring truly is. Because so many clinicians are unaware that postpartum psychosis is, as most researchers believe, a variant of bipolar disorder, they tend to discontinue antipsychotic and mood-stabilizing medications within a year of the episode. Left to her own devices, the woman might either be afraid to conceive again because of a relapse or might fear that if she did become pregnant while taking mood stabilizers—some of which are known to cause birth defects—she would have to terminate the pregnancy.

In fact, medical professionals often discourage women with bipolar disease from attempting to have children. In 2002 a survey of bipolar women seeking prepregnancy advice, done by Dr. Adele Viguera and colleagues and published in the *American Journal of Psychiatry*, found that 45 percent of the seventy responders had been told by a mental health professional to avoid pregnancy altogether. After proper counseling, however, forty-six women decided to pursue pregnancy. Those who chose to avoid pregnancy were fearful of the effects their medication might have on the fetus and were concerned that if they discontinued the medication they would relapse.

One Canadian researcher, Dr. Paul Grof, has suggested, however, that pregnancy has a protective effect for at least one specific group of bipolar patients—those who respond well to lithium—and that a subgroup of these could be managed without mood stabilizers for prolonged periods of time during pregnancy.

Mila, for example, had gone through a severe psychotic episode after the birth of her first child. At the time, she'd been hospitalized, and I'd started her on a combination of Seroquel (quetiapine), an antipsychotic, and the mood stabilizer lithium. After about a year, during which she remained stable, we began to taper her gradually off the lithium because she was planning a second pregnancy. She conceived and continued to remain stable without the lithium. In her third trimester, however, she and her husband came in for a final antenatal consultation, at which time they revealed that her paternal uncle was receiving treatment for bipolar illness and, in addition, her maternal grandmother was in a psychiatric hospital and suspected of having the same disease. With that history, Mila and her husband were extremely concerned that she might relapse in the postpartum period, and we planned that she would restart her lithium on the day she gave birth.

Eighteen months ago as of this writing, Mila had a healthy seven-and-a-half-pound baby girl. She did go back on the lithium immediately and decided not to breast-feed. She is now back at work full time and is extremely grateful that she was able to get through her pregnancy without medication or complications. But in many instances it's impossible for a woman to stop taking her mood stabilizers during pregnancy.

In a study done by Dr. M. C. Blehar and colleagues at the National Institute of Mental Health, 45 percent of those with bipolar disease actually experienced an exacerbation of their illness during pregnancy. Another, done by Dr. Freeman and her group in Tucson, found that 50 percent of their previously stable bipolar subjects became symptomatic during pregnancy. Finally, Dr. Viguera and her colleagues in Boston, studying the risk of recurrence of bipolar disorder in forty-two women who discontinued lithium during pregnancy, found that 52 percent relapsed and that the risk of relapse was increased in those who'd had four or more previous bipolar episodes and discontinued lithium abruptly prior to pregnancy. So it seems that many bipolar women are at very high risk for relapse during pregnancy, particularly if they discontinue their medication.

When she was an adolescent Jules had what in retrospect appears to have been a serious depressive episode followed by a short period of hypomania. At the time, however, she wasn't diagnosed as bipolar, and throughout her twenties she remained symptom free. A gregarious and outgoing young woman as well as a talented pianist, she graduated from business school, and when she was thirty-two years old she moved from Toronto to Vancouver. The following spring she experienced an episode of hypomania that was so serious she required hospitalization.

At first none of Jules's friends could believe she was truly ill because she seemed so happy. For her the tipping point at which a buoyant mood became clinical hypomania was an extremely fine line. But she was, in fact, hospitalized for three months, and when she was discharged the following winter she had a serious depressive disorder. She tried using a light box, but it didn't help, and then in the summer she had another happy spell, which was followed by yet another dark spell. The following summer, when she began to show symptoms of becoming speedy and hyperactive, her family physician decided to treat her with a combination of a mood stabilizer and one of the newer antipsychotics.

Jules did well that year, and she met a gentleman whom she eventually married. When she and her husband came to me for a prenatal consultation Jules was taking lithium, and we decided that she would continue to take her medication and try for a pregnancy. When she conceived, she was taking 600 mg of lithium daily. She did not stop taking her meds, and at sixteen weeks gestation we did a high-resolution ultrasound and performed a fetal echocardiogram. We did an alpha-fetoprotein screening earlier to rule out chromosomal abnormalities. All the results were negative for any defect or problem, and Jules's pregnancy proceeded well until the beginning of the second trimester, when she began to experience fluctuations of mood and became increasingly irritable and hostile. At the time she was the owner of a clothing store, and her employees were becoming concerned about her, so Jules decided to take some time off to "get her head together."

At that point I added one of the newer antipsychotics to the lithium she was already taking, and within two weeks her early delusional symptoms disappeared. She continued to take lithium throughout her pregnancy and postpartum; we monitored her blood levels regularly, reducing the dose a week prior to her giving birth to be sure she didn't become toxic. After delivery, we again increased it in the postpartum period.

I'll be discussing the use of mood stabilizers with bipolar women during pregnancy much more thoroughly in Chapter 8, but for now, I want to make two important points. The first is that it's extremely important to be cognizant of even the most minor mood changes before they become major, and the second is that Jules could not possibly have gotten through her pregnancy without a serious relapse had she not continued to take her medication. And had she not increased her dose of lithium after the birth of her child, there is every indication—both scientifically and anecdotally—that she would have been at serious risk for postpartum psychosis.

The rate of recurrence in the first six months postpartum for women with a previous history of bipolar disease is estimated at anywhere from 20 to 80 percent, and of course the most serious concern when this does occur is for the safety of the infant. Although I've been lucky enough never to have treated a patient who committed infanticide, I have been called as an expert witness in two such cases. One that I will never forget involved Nadia, a young woman with no history of bipolar disorder who became acutely psychotic within three days of giving birth. One aspect of her psychosis was the delusion that her baby was not normal and was not breathing properly. One night, after her husband was asleep, Nadia suffocated the baby in his crib. When I met with her and her husband prior to my testimony, she was distraught, extremely ill, and still totally out of touch with reality.

As with Nadia, the vast majority of psychotic episodes are related to the manic stage of bipolar disease, but in rare instances—as in the tragic case of Andrea Yates, who killed her five children—depression not related to bipolar illness can also be accompanied by delusions and hallucinations. This was the case for the second young woman for whom I was called upon to testify in court. I'd met Yvette while I was traveling to the interior of British Columbia for one of the outreach programs I run at my hospital. At the time she was pregnant and beginning to experience depressive symptoms with paranoid delusions about something being wrong with her baby. We started her on a combination of antidepressants and an antipsychotic without a mood stabilizer. We kept in touch and continued to monitor her until she moved to another, more remote city and we lost contact with her entirely.

Sadly, the next I heard about Yvette was several months later, when I received a phone call from a prosecuting attorney informing me that she had shaken her thirteen-day-old infant because she was no longer able to tolerate the baby's crying and was still convinced that he wasn't normal. When I went to see her in conjunction with my testimony, I was horrified to learn that once she left my care she had stopped taking her medications and had continued to show symptoms of depression and paranoid delusions after the baby's birth.

Whenever we hear of such a tragic case, our tendency is to exclaim, "Who in their right mind would do such a thing?" But, of course, that's just the point—these women are *not* in their right mind. Thankfully, incidents of actual infanticide are as rare as they are shocking. That doesn't mean, however, that any woman experiencing a postnatal psychotic episode couldn't be at risk for performing such an act. The more aware at-risk women are of the possibility, remote though it might be, and the more vigilant health care providers are about monitoring their patients' moods, the less likely it is that depression or bipolar disease will progress to such a point.

PART

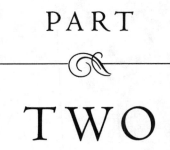

TWO

8

Medicating Depression
During Pregnancy

Antidepressants

The first antidepressant medications were discovered serendipitously when, in the 1950s, patients with tuberculosis (TB) were being treated in sanatoriums, removed from friends and family, and shunned almost like lepers. Quite naturally, many of these patients would have been dejected and depressed, not only by the fact that they were ill but also by their isolation. Their doctors, however, began to notice that patients being treated with the anti-TB drug iproniazid were becoming happy—even euphoric.

As a direct result of this observation, the first tricyclic antidepressant, imipramine, was launched in 1958, revolutionizing the treatment of depression in modern times. Innovations in psychiatry are few and far between. In 1894 Emil Kraepelin, a German psychiatrist, first noted that some patients experienced mood swings, going from extremely depressed to extremely euphoric, and thus identified manic-depression, the illness now known as bipolar disorder. In 1917 Sigmund Freud published *Mourning and Melancholia*, which for the first time explained depression in psychoanalytic terms and identified it as a "disease of the mind."

Then in the 1930s, Drs. Lucio Bini and Ugo Cerletti, two Italian psychiatrists and researchers, performed electroconvulsive therapy for the first time as a treatment for the severely mentally ill. With the advent of imipramine, however, we began to view depression in an entirely different light.

Before we had sophisticated brain imaging techniques such as computed tomography (CT) scans and magnetic resonance imaging (MRI), introduced in the 1970s and 1980s, respectively, there had been no way to see the connection between depression and brain chemistry. But because we knew that imipramine worked by increasing levels of the neurotransmitters norepinephrine and serotonin, that link was now established. As a result, the lives of depressed patients were changed in two ways. Not only were their symptoms significantly alleviated, but they were also seen for the first time—by themselves and others—to be victims of a biochemical imbalance rather than simply as "crazy."

Imipramine, however, was far from perfect. Although it was effective for controlling depression, an overdose could be fatal, and not everyone could tolerate it. For the next few decades researchers and pharmaceutical companies concentrated on developing an antidepressant that would be even more effective and have fewer contraindications. In 1987 Prozac (fluoxetine), introduced by the Eli Lilly company, became almost instantly the world's most successful antidepressant. Prozac, a selective serotonin reuptake inhibitor (SSRI), confirmed the link between serotonin and depression. Since then, many more SSRIs have been developed. Paxil IR and Paxil CR (paroxetine), Zoloft (sertraline), Celexa (citalopram), and Lexapro or Cepralex (escitalopram) are among those that are now most commonly used, but Paxil CR is the only SSRI currently available in controlled-release form. The benefit of controlled-release capsules is that the amount of medication in the system remains steady throughout the day, providing more consistent results and also possibly helping to reduce potential side effects.

Although we are still far from a total understanding of the complex pathways that govern depression, we are making progress year by year. Since the success of the SSRIs, dual-action antidepressants—serotonin and norepinephrine reuptake inhibitors (SNRIs) and noradrenergic and specific serotonergic antidepressants (NaSSAs)—have taken us yet a step further. SNRIs prevent the reabsorption of both noradrenaline and serotonin. At the moment Effexor XR (venlafaxine) is the only one of this class of antidepressants available in sustained-release capsule form. NaSSAs increase the release of noradrenaline in certain areas of the brain and target specific serotonin receptors, thereby enhancing its production. Remeron (mirtazapine) belongs to this class of drugs. Atypical antidepressant Wellbutrin (bupropion) acts on dopamine and norepinephrine neurotransmitters.

The goal, of course, for each new drug is to improve upon the efficacy and safety of the previous class by acting more specifically, more quickly, and with fewer side effects.

Table 1. CLASSIFICATIONS OF ANTIDEPRESSANTS

Class	Generic Name	Brand Names	Dose (mg/day)
Tricyclic antidepressants (TCAs)			
	Amitriptyline	Elavil; Endep; Emitrip; Levate; Novotriptyn	150–300
	Clomipramine	Anafranil	150–250
	Desipramine	Norpramin; Pertofrane	150–300
	Doxepin	Sinequan; Adapin; Zonalon; Triadaprin	150–300
	Imipramine	Tofranil; Janimine; Norfranil; Tipramine; Impril; Novapramine	150–300
	Nortriptyline	Aventyl; Pamelor; Allegron	75–150
	Trimipramine	Surmontil; Rhotrimine	75–300
Monoamine oxidase inhibitors (MAOIs)			
	Isocarboxazid	Marplan	30–60
	Phenelzine	Nardil	45–90
	Tranylcypromine	Parnate	30–60
Reversible MAOIs			
	Moclobemide	Manerix	300–600

Selective serotonin reuptake inhibitors (SSRIs)

Fluoxetine	Prozac; Lorien; Lovan; Zactin; Erocap	20–60
Paroxetine	Paxil; Seroxat; Aropax; Lumin	20–50
Citalopram	Celexa; Cipramil	20–60
Sertraline	Zoloft; Lustral	50–200
Escitalopram	Lexapro; Cepralex	20–40
Fluvoxamine	Luvox; Faverin	50–300

Atypical antidepressants

Buproprion	Wellbutrin; Zyban; Amfebutamone	150–450
Trazodone	Desyrel; Trazon; Trialodine; Molipaxin	200–300

Noradrenergic and specific serotonergic antidepressants (NaSSAs)

Mirtazapine	Remeron; Avanza	15–45

Serotonin norepinephrine reuptake inhibitors (SNRIs)

Venlafaxine	Effexor	150–375

Antidepressants and Pregnancy: The Dilemma of Exposure

By trying to minimize the exposure of the fetus to medication and, at the same time, limit the fetal risks of untreated depression, the clinician is, as Dr. Lee Cohen of Harvard Medical School has put it, caught between "a teratologic rock and a clinical hard place." A teratogen can be any substance that has the potential to cause birth defects or congenital malformations in animals or humans, and, as we learned only too tragically with thalidomide, drugs that may be safe for use in animals during pregnancy may have a very different effect in humans.

Yet we've been treating pregnant women successfully with antidepressants for more than forty years. In fact, given that more than half the pregnancies in the United States are unplanned, fetal exposure to medication—particularly to antidepressant medication—is bound to occur before the woman or her doctor realizes that she's pregnant. In addition, statistics as reported in 2003 in the *Current Women's Health Report* indicate that up to 80 percent of women take prescribed medications during pregnancy, and of those, 35 percent are taking psychotropic medications.

Not surprisingly, of the psychotropic drugs taken during pregnancy, antidepressants are those for which we've accumulated the most data. I say "not surprisingly" because, as we've seen, depression is one of the most common illnesses suffered by women of childbearing age, and despite the widespread cultural myths describing pregnancy and childbirth as among the happiest times in a woman's life, the truth is that up to 70 percent of pregnant women experience some degree of depressive symptoms during pregnancy, and of those, 12 percent meet the diagnostic criteria for major depression.

A recent study funded by the National Institute of Mental Health and conducted by Dr. Lee Cohen of Harvard Medical School, Dr. Lori Altshuler of the University of California at Los Angeles, and Dr. Zack Stowe of Emory University identified fifty-four women with a history of major depression who elected to discontinue antidepressant therapy either prior to or immediately after conception. The investigators observed the women throughout their pregnancies and, not surprisingly, found that twenty-three of the fifty-four (42 percent) relapsed—eleven in the first trimester, eight in the second, and four in the third, thus challenging previous assumptions about the protective effects of pregnancy.

According to Dr. Jack Gorman of the Mount Sinai School of Medicine in New York City:

> Pregnancy is often described as a time of emotional bliss. Morning sickness and other physical discomfort not withstanding, pregnant women are traditionally said to "glow," euphoric about the impending addition to their lives. No doubt, this description was concocted by men. Although most women are perhaps happy to be pregnant, many are not. These include teenagers and women beset with overwhelming financial and social problems. For such women, having a baby may not represent life's ultimate fulfillment. Other women

worry about the effect of a new baby on their careers. Some obsess about whether they will make a good mother. For whatever reason, pregnancy can be an enormously stressful and, for a minority, a harrowing time of life.

Despite the risks—and, indeed, there are risks—of taking antidepressant medication, the outcome of untreated depression can, as we've already seen and as I'll be discussing further in the chapters that follow, be quite serious if not devastating for both mother and fetus. In fact, Dr. Stowe calls the havoc created by an untreated chemical imbalance during pregnancy the "first adverse event" in the life of the fetus.

For many women as well as many physicians, the instinctive reaction to pregnancy is to reduce or abruptly stop taking antidepressants. But this well-meaning attempt to limit fetal exposure actually increases the woman's risk of relapsing and thus the likelihood that both she and her fetus will be exposed to the illness as well as to the medication.

Given what we know of the consequences, untreated or undertreated depression is, in my opinion, a far more dangerous teratogen than pharmacological treatment. But that is a decision each woman must make for herself in conjunction with her physician. And that is why I'm hoping, with this book, to help her make a decision that is based upon informed consent rather than fear.

Informed Consent

In the end, every woman is the captain of her own ship. Only she can ultimately decide whether or not she will take medication, which is why it's so very important that she be as educated as possible about the options, their possible risks, and their potential benefits. The more a woman is able to feel that she is a participating partner in her treatment program, the more likely she will be to comply with and follow through on the plan.

Therefore, any woman who is planning to become pregnant and is either taking antidepressant medication or has a history of depression (even if she is not currently taking medication) should consult with her psychiatrist prior to conception.

If you are reading this and fit into one of those categories, you will probably have questions about one or more of the following issues:

- The risks of prenatal exposure to antidepressants
- The risk of relapse if you discontinue your medication
- The impact of untreated depression on your own well-being as well as that of your baby
- The risk of relapse in the postpartum period and the possibility of preventative postpartum treatment
- The role of nonpharmacological treatment in your particular case

When Pharmacological Treatment Is the Right Choice

In my opinion and experience, pharmacological therapy is indicated if:

- A woman is suffering a moderate to severe degree of depression during pregnancy.
- A woman is contemplating pregnancy and prior attempts to discontinue medications have failed.
- A woman relapses with depressive symptoms during pregnancy.
- A woman has a family history of psychiatric illness and is therefore at high risk of a new depressive episode during pregnancy.
- A woman has preexisting symptoms of OCD, panic disorder, or another psychiatric diagnosis with accompanying depression that increases during pregnancy.

If you fit into any of these categories, if your depression is currently interfering with your well-being, if you've already experienced recurrent depression, and especially if you've ever experienced symptoms severe enough to have been psychotic or suicidal, I would suggest that you have virtually no option but to continue your medication during pregnancy.

After consulting with your physician and assessing the risks, however, you will still have to find the best medication for your situation and symptoms, and that in itself can be a challenge. There are presently more than fifty different medications available, so the goal is to find the one that provides the most relief with the fewest side effects.

Research indicates that almost half of all patients stop taking their antidepressant medication within the first month because of adverse side effects. Generally speaking, it takes four to six weeks to confirm that a medication is effective, and in most cases the patient will experience side effects before she sees any positive effect, which makes it difficult to convince her to stick with it. The good news, however, is that more than 80 percent of those who do stick with it will respond positively to at least one medication.

Currently SSRIs are the medications most commonly used for pregnant and postpartum women, although in the past few years the use of Effexor (venlafaxine), an SNRI, seems to be steadily increasing as well. Previously, tricyclic antidepressants were shown to be quite effective, but their troublesome and uncomfortable side effects (which might include constipation, blurred vision, stomach upsets, hypotension, effects on the heart, and even the risk of death if the patient takes an overdose) have always been an issue, and for that reason their use is now limited in pregnancy and postpartum, the newer medications being much safer by comparison.

The American Psychiatric Association's Committee on Research on Psychiatric Treatments has identified depression during pregnancy as a priority for improved clinical practice. The problem, however, is that the Food and Drug Administration's classification of drugs for teratogenic risk is not adequate to address the issue of taking antidepressants during pregnancy and does not provide adequate guidance for clinicians. A particularly telling example of this is the FDA and Health Canada warning that third-trimester exposure to either SSRIs or SNRIs could lead to neonatal complications. We know that depression does not get better in the last trimester; in fact, it actually gets worse. So reducing the dose or stopping medication is sure to lead to relapse. In light of the FDA and Health Canada warning, what are clinicians and patients to think? The frustrating facts are that this warning is based on very small studies, case reports, and retrospective data and that it may cause conflict for the clinician with clinical observation of the significance of maternal mental illness in the third trimester for both mother and baby.

In light of the confusion caused by the FDA and Health Canada classifications, many researchers and clinicians have recommended that they be replaced by statements and summaries of currently available data regarding the fetal risk attendant upon each medication. At present, the FDA rates medications as falling into one of five risk categories—A, B, C, D, and X—A meaning safe for use during pregnancy and X meaning that the drug has proved to be unsafe. Most psychotropic medications are classified C, meaning that risk cannot be ruled out.

U.S. FOOD AND DRUG ADMINISTRATION (FDA) USE-IN-PREGNANCY RATINGS	
Category	*Interpretation*
A	**Controlled studies show no risk.** Adequate well-controlled studies in pregnant women have failed to demonstrate risk to the fetus.
B	**No evidence of risk in humans.** Either animal findings show risk but human findings do not, or if no adequate human studies have been done, animal findings are negative.
C	**Risk cannot be ruled out.** Human studies are lacking, and animal studies are either positive for fetal risk or lacking as well; however, potential benefits may justify potential risk.
D	**Positive evidence of risk.** Investigational or postmarketing data show risk to the fetus; nevertheless, potential benefits may outweigh risks.
X	**Contraindicated in pregnancy.** Studies in animals or humans, or investigational or postmarketing reports, have shown fetal risks that clearly outweigh any possible benefit to the patient.

At the moment, therefore, all use of psychotropic medications, including antidepressants, during pregnancy is considered "off-label," meaning that their use in pregnant and lactating women is not officially indicated or sanctioned. There are, however, ways to minimize the risk of drug exposure during the sensitive periods of pregnancy. These include:

- Using the lowest possible dose to achieve therapeutic response
- Choosing, whenever possible, to use a medication that is known to result in low possible fetal or neonatal exposure
- Seeking the medication that may have minimal effects on the newborn
- Avoiding newer medications unless there is a body of information regarding the effects of their use during human pregnancy

That said, however, if a woman has been doing well on one of the newer medications, such as Celexa, it would be unwise to switch. Changing medications is likely to result in relapse and would also expose mother and fetus to two medications rather than one, thus jeopardizing the health of both mother and child.

The Risks of Fetal Exposure

In order to understand how any medication may affect the developing fetus, it's necessary to have some knowledge of how that development proceeds. Organogenesis (the development of the baby in utero) occurs in the following order:

0 to 4 weeks: Fertilization occurs; the embryo travels through the fallopian tubes and implants in the uterine wall; the nervous system, brain, digestive system, ears, and arms begin to form; the heart forms and begins to beat at twenty-one days.

5 to 8 weeks: The nostrils, eyelids, nose, fingers, legs, feet, toes, and bones begin to form; females develop ovaries, males develop testes; the head is as large as the body; the cardiovascular system is fully functional.

9 to 12 weeks: The embryo becomes a fetus (from eight weeks until birth, the developing child is called a fetus); the penis makes males distinct; growth of the chin and other facial structures give the fetus a human face and profile.

13 to 16 weeks: Blinking of eyes and sucking of lips occur; the body begins to outgrow the head; the mother can feel the muscular activity of the fetus, such as kicking.

17 to 20 weeks: The limbs achieve their final proportions; eyelashes and eyebrows have formed.

21 to 30 weeks: There is a substantial increase in weight; the fetus may survive if born at this point; the skin is wrinkled and red.

30 to 40 weeks: The fingernails and toenails have developed.

The reason it's important to be aware of this calendar of fetal development is that if malformations do occur, this happens when the organs are being formed—that is, during the first four weeks of pregnancy. Discontinuing medication would, therefore, make sense only if the pregnancy is confirmed during the first two weeks after conception, but very few women can be sure they are pregnant at that early date. After that point, the next time we are concerned about fetal exposure is during the third trimester because of possible toxicity in the newborn. In the pages that follow, I'll be discussing the monitoring of antidepressant dosages at each stage of pregnancy as well as in the postpartum period. First, however, I'd like to pass along some of the most current research into the risks of fetal exposure to various types of medication and what we've been able to find out.

Placental Passage of Antidepressant Medications

The placenta is the tissue through which the fetus receives from the mother all the nutrients that sustain it throughout the pregnancy. This means, however, that other substances, including medications, may also be transferred by the mother to the child she is carrying, which is why we're concerned about fetal exposure to antidepressants.

Researchers have studied the ways various antidepressants travel across the placenta. In one such study, Dr. Victoria Hendrick and her colleagues looked at thirty-eight pregnant women who were exposed to Celexa, Prozac, Paxil, or Zoloft. Measuring the levels of medication in the umbilical cord, through which they are transferred to the fetus, and comparing them with maternal blood levels, the researchers found that the ratios were lower for Zoloft and Paxil than they were for Prozac and Celexa. The significance of these findings, however, remains to be determined. Not only are there various factors that could influence the passage of medication across the placenta, but also the risk involved in the higher levels of one drug rather than another is at this time still open to question.

The research group at my own hospital has conducted a similar study, measuring levels of Paxil, Prozac, and Zoloft in the maternal blood during pregnancy, in the umbilical cord at delivery, and in the infant's blood two days after delivery. We found that the concentrations of Prozac and its metabolite norfluoxetine were higher in the maternal blood as well as in the infant than were concentrations of Paxil or Zoloft, thus confirming Dr. Hendrick's findings and determining that infant exposure to Prozac was probably higher than it was to either Paxil or Zoloft. However, when we measured the levels of the same medications two months later, this difference did not exist.

What both these studies indicate is that all of the medications we monitored were transferred through the umbilical cord to the placenta, although to varying degrees. Knowing that, every woman needs to weigh the risks, insofar as we know them, of taking antidepressant medications both during pregnancy and in the postpartum period against the risks of discontinuing medication or refusing it should she become depressed after conception.

To help you do that, I've already indicated that if you are depressed, you will not be physically or mentally healthy enough to go through the entire forty weeks of pregnancy, and in Chapter 11 I'll talk more directly about the additional risks to which you will be exposing the fetus. Now, so that you will be more aware of your options with regard to antidepressant medications and how each of them may affect both you and your child, I'll provide what information we have about the risk/benefit ratios of each class of drug.

At this point, it's important to note that all available studies on each of these medications have been done using the brand-name compound, not generic drugs. For this reason, I would urge any woman taking antidepressants to stick with the brand even though it is more expensive. Although generics are meant to be identical to the original branded drug, we do not, for example, know what materials are used in the coatings or capsules, and they may also differ from one manufacturer to another. So the safety data that has been accumulated on the branded product cannot at this point necessarily be applied to generics.

The Risks and Benefits of Antidepressant Medications

SELECTIVE SEROTONIN REUPTAKE INHIBITORS (SSRIs)
Prozac (fluoxetine)

Four prospective or long-term studies have evaluated more than 1,500 infants exposed to fluoxetine and have found no increase in the incidence of malformation. A paper by Dr. C. D. Chambers published in the *New England Journal of Medicine* in 1996 described three minor anomalies, but these have not been replicated in subsequent studies, and Dr. Chambers's study has come under criticism for other reasons, including the fact that it did not take into account the effect of maternal mood on the baby's outcome. So at this time fluoxetine is not considered to be a teratogen.

This is also one medication for which we have information on long-term effects of exposure in utero. A study done by Dr. I. Nulman and colleagues of the Motherisk program in Toronto and published in the *New England Journal of Medicine* in 1997 followed fifty-five mother-infant pairs between sixteen and eighty-six months (seven years) after exposure to fluoxetine and reported no differences in general IQ levels or in language or behavioral development as compared both to those exposed to tricyclic antidepressants and to those who had been exposed to no medication at all. In another follow-up study published in the

American Journal of Psychiatry in 2002, the same researchers studied forty-six infants who had been exposed to fluoxetine during pregnancy up to seventy-one months (six years) after birth and found that they had been in no way compromised in terms of cognition or language ability. They did find, on the other hand, that the duration of maternal depression and the number of depressive episodes the mother experienced after birth correlated to lower cognition and language achievement in their children. So again, the degree of maternal depression appeared to have a greater impact on child development than did the baby's exposure to fluoxetine.

A word of caution, however. Just because Prozac has been studied more widely than other SSRIs and has been shown to be safe, it would be wrong to assume that this would necessarily be the drug of choice for everyone. If a woman has taken Prozac in the past and has not responded positively, or if she is responding well either to another SSRI or to Effexor when she becomes pregnant, changing medications could be a big mistake, as it was for Dana, who became a patient of mine after she'd switched from Effexor to Prozac.

Dana had been taking 225 mg of Effexor for about four years and her symptoms were in complete remission when, at the age of forty-two, she inadvertently conceived. Because she was familiar with the literature on Prozac, she decided on her own to abruptly stop taking her Effexor. Within three weeks her depressive symptoms returned, and she went to see her family physician. Together they decided that she would then begin taking Prozac. She started with a dose of 20 mg and went up to 40 mg and then to 60 with no resolution of her symptoms. By the time she arrived in my office she was twenty-one weeks pregnant, and her baby had by then been exposed to both Effexor (before she realized she'd conceived) and Prozac. After consulting with my colleagues, we determined that she should stop taking Prozac and go back on Effexor, which had been effective for her in the past. Even so, her symptoms did not remit until after she'd given birth, and in the postpartum period we had to increase her Effexor to 300 mg—much more than she'd been taking during pregnancy—in order for her to achieve emotional stability.

In Dana's case, the fact that she'd been in remission and emotionally healthy on Effexor far outweighed the possible effects the medication might have had on her baby. In addition, by the time she realized she was pregnant, the fetus had already been exposed to the drug. So changing her medication meant not only that she became sicker but also that her baby was being exposed to two antidepressants rather than just one, and whatever congenital malformation (if any) Effexor might have caused would already have taken place. Luckily, this didn't happen. Dana's baby was born full-term, completely healthy, and with absolutely no symptoms of withdrawal.

Paxil (paroxetine)

To date, there have been no reports at all of increased rates of major anatomical or physical malformations, stillbirths, miscarriages, or prematurity associated with the use of paroxetine during pregnancy. One study, conducted by Nathalie Kulin and colleagues at the Motherisk Program, looked at 267 women exposed to SSRIs, including 97 who took paroxetine, and compared them to a control group. Their findings indicated that first-trimester exposure to paroxetine was risk free. We have data on 247 pregnancies on Paxil.

In terms of neonatal toxicity, one study, which has been criticized for its methodology, has reported neonatal withdrawal symptoms including jitteriness, jaundice, and hypoglycemia. Our own study, however, found no symptoms of withdrawal in babies who had been exposed to Paxil alone but did find that when it was combined with Klonopin (clonazepam), an anticonvulsant medication also prescribed to alleviate anxiety, the probability of withdrawal was increased. In fact, we had in our study one woman who had been receiving 60 mg of Paxil—a high dose—and we were concerned enough to have a neonatologist on alert at the time she gave birth, but the baby showed no signs of withdrawal whatsoever.

Another study, conducted by Dr. B. Kallen in Sweden, followed 106 women taking Paxil throughout their pregnancy and determined that neonatal toxicity was not of particular concern. Dr. Kallen also looked at 997 infants who had been exposed to antidepressants during late pregnancy. Of these, 558 had been exposed to SSRIs—285 to Celexa, 106 to Paxil, 91 to Prozac, and 77 to Zoloft. His conclusion was that there was no difference between Paxil and the other SSRIs in terms of neonatal complications.

The point to remember here is that there are many factors determining whether or not an infant will experience withdrawal from any medication. These might include the way the medication is absorbed and distributed in the mother's blood, the way it is metabolized by both mother and fetus, and the way it is eliminated by the baby's liver. At this point, most researchers agree that it is important to investigate factors beyond the medication itself that could contribute to neonatal toxicity. Those factors might be premature birth, low birth weight, whether or not the mother smoked cigarettes or drank alcohol, and whether or not she was taking other medications during pregnancy. However, the most important factor of all with relation to poor neonatal outcome is the severity of the illness itself. My colleagues and I have recently published a study in which we found that the mothers of babies who demonstrated poor neonatal adaptation were severely depressed and suffered from comorbid anxiety disorders (at least one anxiety disorder that existed concurrently with a depressive episode). Of the forty-six babies included in the study, eleven needed to be in an intensive care nursery for respiratory support. Happily, however, all these babies recovered completely within twenty-four to forty-eight hours and went home healthy with their mothers. Our findings suggest that maternal psychiatric status is a critical variable that influences infant outcome.

In my opinion, therefore, it would be unwise for anyone to stop taking a medication that was helping her because she was worried about neonatal toxicity. Even if "poor neonatal adaptation" symptoms do occur, our experience indicates that they are transient in nature, do not have long-term effects on the baby, and can be treated effectively in a hospital setting.

With regard to neurobehavioral effects over the long term in babies who'd had prenatal exposure to SSRIs, we looked at a total of twenty-two children—fourteen exposed to Paxil, five to Prozac, and three to Zoloft—four years after birth and compared them to a control group; we found no differences in the children's mood, behavior, and emotional responses between the exposed group and the nonexposed group. In fact, because chronic relapsing depression in mothers parenting their newborns up to four years of age does seem to have a negative impact on some aspects of the children's behavior (i.e., their emotions, withdrawal, and irritability), my recommendation at this time is to treat the maternal depression when it is diagnosed in pregnancy.

Zoloft (sertraline)

Given what information we've gathered so far, there is no data to indicate that Zoloft is associated with either congenital malformation or impaired neurological development. In Dr. Kulin's study, cited on page 157, there were 147 women who had been exposed to Zoloft, all of whose babies were born with no malformation. A total of 226 reports on Zoloft pregnancy have been reported. And in our own prospective study of four-year-olds, there was no indication of impaired language or cognitive development, emotional problems, hyperactivity, or aggression. Presently, there have been a few reports of withdrawal symptoms, but the numbers are small.

Celexa (citalopram)

The Swedish birth registry study reported by Dr. Erikson documented approximately 365 cases of women who had used Celexa during pregnancy with no apparent risk to the newborn. To date, there have been no long-term studies and therefore no data available on the potential for impaired neurological development in children who were exposed to this particular medication in utero.

SEROTONIN AND NOREPINEPHRINE REUPTAKE INHIBITORS (SNRIs)

Effexor (venlafaxine)

The use of Effexor has increased considerably in the recent past, possibly because it is associated with high remission rates in depression. At my clinic, therefore, we are encountering many women who either already were taking Effexor when they got pregnant or for whom it is being prescribed during pregnancy because they have not responded well to a previous medication.

Another Motherisk study, this one conducted in 2001 by Dr.

Adrienne Einarson, a well-known researcher with nursing credentials, and colleagues, included 150 women who had been exposed to Effexor during the first trimester of their pregnancy. The study did not show any increase in birth defects among this group, and to date there are no neonatal toxic symptoms associated with its use. Because it is relatively new on the market, however, there has not yet been time for long-term studies to assess its potential for causing developmental neurological impairment.

Currently, Effexor is being included in a study I'm conducting with my colleague Dr. Tim Oberlander in collaboration with the March of Dimes and Yale University on the effects of exposure to various psychotropic medications during pregnancy and lactation. For now, however, when patients ask whether it's worse to take one of these newer medications than it would be to take an older one, my response has to be that there is not yet sufficient data available to answer that question, but the data we do have on older medications are reassuring, and it would be best for them to stick to whichever medication has been most effective for them. In other words, if they've been taking one of the newer medications and it's been working for them, they shouldn't stop taking it during pregnancy just because it's new.

TRICYCLIC ANTIDEPRESSANTS (TCAs)

Because tricyclic antidepressants have been around for a long time, we have documentation of more than four hundred cases involving women who were exposed to them during their first trimester. The data indicates that Anafranil (clomipramine) in particular has been associated with neonatal toxicity in the form of mild respiratory distress, tremors, and jitteriness as well as other toxic symptoms, all of which, however, have been transitory, lasting no more than twenty-four to forty-eight hours.

Long-term studies of babies exposed to TCAs in utero have shown no differences three years later in IQ, language, temperament, or mood when compared to children who were not exposed.

Among the TCAs, Norpramin and Pertofrane (desipramine) and Aventyl, Pamelor, and Allegron (nortriptyline) are generally preferred to Anafranil (clomipramine) because they have fewer sedative, gastro-intestinal, cardiac, and hypotensive side effects. Generally speaking, how-ever, their side effects remain more troublesome than those associated with SSRIs, and for that reason they are now rarely used as the drug of choice for treatment of depression. That said, however, when you are determining what drug you feel comfortable taking during pregnancy, you must weigh the potential discomfort of possible side effects against the relative comfort you might derive from taking a medication about which there is abundant published data.

I recently worked with a patient who had been in remission and well maintained on 200 mg of Zoloft, but when she became pregnant she in-sisted that she wanted to discontinue her Zoloft and switch to Pertofrane (a TCA) instead. She experienced dry mouth and felt extraordinarily sedated while taking Pertofrane—symptoms she had not experienced with Zoloft—but said that the side effects were worth it to her because she felt more comfortable taking a medication whose safety data were well established.

Then, after she gave birth and wanted to breast-feed her baby, she determined to go back to Zoloft because she knew that studies had indi-cated it was a safe medication to take while nursing.

At that point, I had to let her know that if our goal was to keep her mood stable while putting her baby at the least possible risk, it seemed unwise to me to expose him to a second drug during lactation. In the end, however, after offering my professional opinion as a clinician, I had to support her in her decision. In this case, we monitored her closely and there were no problems, but I would still caution against exposing a fetus or infant to more than one medication. As I've said, when it comes to decisions concerning antidepressant medication, a woman is the cap-tain of her ship. Except in the most extreme circumstances, we can't force anyone to take medication, and it is therefore important to make the patient an ally who willingly "follows the program," so to speak, rather than risk losing her cooperation or having her abandon treat-ment entirely.

OTHER ANTIDEPRESSANTS

Of the remaining antidepressants currently available, Remeron (mirtazapine), Wellbutrin (bupropion), and Desyrel (trazodone) need to be mentioned, although the information we have on them so far is quite limited. GlaxoSmithKline now has a registry of 534 women taking Wellbutrin during the first trimester of pregnancy with no increase in birth defects. For Remeron there are only nine case reports, but all of them have resulted in healthy babies with no apparent toxicity. Desyrel, the third of these atypical antidepressants, is rarely used alone; generally it is prescribed in combination with other antidepressants. Of the fifty-eight reports we have of its use during pregnancy, none has shown any increase in birth defects.

Administering Antidepressants, Trimester by Trimester

As I've said, the concerns related to taking antidepressant medication depend on the particular stage of the pregnancy. If you are planning a pregnancy, it would be wise to consult with your health care provider prior to conception so that:

- She or he can evaluate your present condition and prior history, make recommendations regarding the use of antidepressants, and monitor you from the start.
- She or he can discuss with you any teratogenic risks associated with your medication and/or discuss its safety in the third trimester.
- She or he can switch you to a safer medication, if necessary, prior to conception.
- Your obstetrician and psychiatrist can coordinate your care.

The following summary is designed to help women and their health care providers deal with any concerns they may have as pregnancy progresses and in the postpartum period.

THE FIRST TRIMESTER

- Educate yourself and be sure that you have not only a strong network of social support but also the support of your caregivers. You will need to be closely monitored with regular follow-up visits to your caregiver from this point on.

- Discuss with your physician any concerns you might have about the teratogenic effects of various medications. At present they appear to be minimal, especially with relation to SSRIs and SNRIs.

- Do not discontinue medication if you have been taking it prior to conception. The medication will ensure that your pregnancy continues safely and uneventfully.

- Make sure that your obstetrician or family doctor is aware of your medication history.

- If you require additional nonpharmacological treatment such as psychotherapy, it should be used in conjunction with your medication.

- If you discontinue medication and choose psychotherapy while pregnant, make sure you are closely monitored.

- If you were not taking antidepressant medication at the time of conception but are aware of symptoms of depression appearing or reappearing, make your doctor aware of them immediately. These symptoms, as we've seen, may be similar to and confused with those of pregnancy, but if there is any doubt in your mind that what you're experiencing is normal, you need to alert your physician.

THE SECOND TRIMESTER

- Be aware that the baby's organs have already been formed during the first trimester.

- If your symptoms become worse, you and your doctor should discuss the need to start you on medication if you are not already taking one or to increase the dose of medication you are already taking.

THE THIRD TRIMESTER

- Although some clinicians may want to decrease the amount of anti-depressant medication a patient is taking in the third trimester to avoid the risk of neonatal withdrawal, my own clinical experience indicates that this is when depressive symptoms are most likely to increase and, as blood volume increases and liver metabolism changes at this time, some women need to increase their doses. In addition, if withdrawal does occur, the symptoms are transient and easily treated in the hospital. As noted earlier, the FDA and Health Canada advisory issued with relation to SSRIs and SNRIs in the third trimester scared a lot of our patients by warning them of the possibility of withdrawal symptoms in newborns. However, it also advises patients to discuss the risk/benefit ratio with their doctors.

- The one exception to this rule is benzodiazepines such as Klonopin and Ativan, which I'll be discussing later in this chapter. Because they are known to be addictive, I always try to get my patients to taper off and, if possible, discontinue benzodiazepines during the third trimester.

- If you are taking more than one medication, discuss with your physician the need to have a neonatologist present at the time of delivery to address any withdrawal symptoms should they occur.

THE POSTPARTUM PERIOD

Any woman with a history of depression has up to a 30 percent risk of relapsing postpartum.

- If you have been taking antidepressants during pregnancy, you need to continue taking them.

- If you have a history of depression—especially recurrent episodes—but were not taking medication during pregnancy, do not wait and see if your symptoms return. I strongly recommend treatment with medication to prevent relapse at this time.

Mood Stabilizers, Anticonvulsants, Antipsychotics, and Antianxiety Medications

Lithium, the First Mood Stabilizer

The oldest of the mood stabilizers, lithium is still one of the medications most commonly used to control bipolar disorder. It was discovered in the late 1800s when doctors who were using the drug to treat patients with gout realized that it had a mood-stabilizing effect. In 1949 Dr. John Cade, an Australian psychiatrist, found that it had calming properties when administered to guinea pigs, and he published a paper outlining its use for the treatment of bipolar disorder. In 1970 it was approved for that use by the Food and Drug Administration, giving hope for the first time to chronic sufferers. But it was not until 1990 that researchers at the University of Wisconsin discovered how it achieved its effect—by working on glutamate, a particular neurotransmitter in the brain.

LITHIUM AND PREGNANCY: ASSESSING THE RISKS

In the early days of lithium's use the International Registry of Lithium Babies indicated that there was a 400-fold increase in the risk of a particular heart defect, Ebstein's anomaly, associated with a woman taking lithium during the first trimester of pregnancy.

More recently, however, Dr. Lee Cohen at Harvard Medical School, in what is, I believe, one of the studies most responsible for decreasing fear of lithium use during pregnancy, analyzed all the reports of Ebstein's anomaly and determined that the risk was lower than previously believed. Dr. Cohen found that it actually occurred in one to two lithium pregnancies per thousand, while in the general population it occurs at the rate of one in twenty thousand live births. This means that the risk for lithium users is increased by 0.1 to 0.05 percent, which is 20 to 40 times higher than the general population but nowhere near the frightening 400-fold we had originally thought.

Any woman who has been exposed to lithium should have a thorough prenatal screening, including a high-resolution ultrasound with echocardiogram of the fetus, at between sixteen and eighteen weeks of gestation. If Ebstein's anomaly is detected at that time, the woman may choose to terminate her pregnancy. In mild form the defect is operable and correctable, but in some cases it may not be compatible with life.

In the second and third trimesters of pregnancy, when the organs have been formed, the risks of lithium exposure are much less significant. There is an extremely small risk that the baby may be hypothyroid, a condition that disappears without treatment. Even rarer is nephrogenic diabetes insipidus, a kidney condition that leaves patients thirsty and dehydrated. And some newborns may experience transitory symptoms of toxicity or "floppy baby syndrome," which is characterized by cyanosis (which causes the baby's skin to appear blue), low muscle tone, lethargy, irritability, and jitteriness—all of which resolve themselves in twenty-four to forty-eight hours with no lasting effect.

To date there have been two studies of the behavioral outcomes of babies exposed to lithium. The first followed sixty children up to five years of age, and the second compared twenty-two lithium-exposed children to a nonexposed control group. Neither study found any behavioral problems associated with lithium exposure.

MATERNAL MONITORING

Maternal hypothyroidism and kidney damage are two potential complications of long-term lithium exposure. Women who are planning a pregnancy should therefore be tested to establish a baseline thyroid function level and should then be tested for thyroid-stimulating hormone concentration during pregnancy. Kidney function should also be tested prior to a woman initiating lithium treatment and should be monitored with blood tests periodically thereafter.

Pregnant women may also occasionally experience polydipsia (increased thirst) and polyuria (excessive urination). While both these symptoms are common in all pregnant women, they may be exacerbated by lithium use.

Some women may also feel sleepy or sedated or may experience tremors, indicating that their lithium levels are too high and their dosage should be adjusted.

It's always important to drink plenty of fluids so that the lithium will be efficiently flushed from the system and to maintain a normal diet so that salt levels remain stable and you don't become dehydrated. Any dietary change that either increases or decreases salt levels can affect blood levels of lithium and should not be undertaken without first consulting with your doctor.

HOW PREGNANCY AFFECTS LITHIUM LEVELS

As pregnancy advances, the kidneys begin to eliminate lithium from the system more quickly, so during the second and third trimesters the dosage may have to be increased in order to maintain the same levels.

During labor and delivery, however, there is a rapid decrease in the filtration of lithium through the kidneys, while at the same time, a substantial amount of fluid is lost by the mother. When these changes occur, lithium levels can increase rapidly, sometimes to toxic levels, in both the mother and the newborn.

Many physicians, therefore, reduce lithium dosage before delivery, but if it is reduced too much—especially if the woman has a long-standing history or frequent episodes of bipolar disorder—she may be at risk for relapse. Dr. Lee Cohen has also studied the risk/benefit ratio of fetal exposure to lithium, and he has found minimal evidence of toxicity in newborns whose mothers received lithium during pregnancy as well as during labor and delivery. My own clinical experience has been that if lithium must be discontinued, it should be done slowly, over a period of time, in order to minimize the risk of relapse.

When we treat women with bipolar disorder who wish to become pregnant, we must weigh the risks of taking psychotropic medications against the potentially negative impact the untreated disorder might have on both the woman and her fetus. Although there is no hard data available on the effects lack of treatment might have on fetal development, we do know that women with untreated bipolar disorder are prone to substance abuse, which can in turn lead to impulsive, aggressive behavior. And without treatment there is always the risk of a patient relapsing and becoming violent or suicidal. Many bipolar women will also fail to seek adequate prenatal care, which could lead to behaviors that are unhealthy for them as well as their babies.

Anyone who does decide to discontinue her lithium during pregnancy should also know that it is imperative for her to resume taking the medication immediately after she gives birth in order to prevent a postpartum relapse. For unmedicated pregnant bipolar patients, the risk of postpartum relapse is close to 70 percent.

GUIDELINES FOR DECIDING WHETHER TO
TAKE LITHIUM DURING PREGNANCY

- Always plan your pregnancy in consultation with your physician.

- Whether or not to continue taking lithium during pregnancy is a decision that must be made on the basis of each woman's personal history of bipolar disorder.

- Anyone who decides to take lithium should have her blood levels monitored regularly throughout pregnancy as well as the postpartum period. Blood levels of lithium should be between 0.621 and 1.2 mEq/L (milliequivalents per liter of blood). Toxicity occurs at levels above 1.2 mEq/L.

- Lithium should be taken in two doses that are separated in time so that levels remain even throughout the day. High-resolution ultrasound between sixteen to eighteen weeks with fetal echocardiogram is recommended.

- Anyone who decides to discontinue lithium during pregnancy must be sure to reinstate it immediately after delivery to avoid a postpartum manic or depressive episode.

- Pregnancy in women taking lithium is classified as high-risk, but it can be managed successfully if treatment is properly planned and monitored closely throughout.

- Whatever her decision with regard to medication, no woman should judge herself harshly. There are no rights or wrongs here, and the ultimate goal is to preserve the patient's mental health while also ensuring a healthy outcome for the baby.

Anticonvulsant Medications

In addition to lithium, many bipolar patients are treated with anticonvulsant medications, which act as mood stabilizers. The most common include:

> Depakote (valproic acid)
> Tegretol (carbamazepine)
> Lamictal (lamotrigine)
> Neurontin (gabapentin)
> Topamax (topiramate)

The bulk of the data we have concerning the use of anticonvulsants during pregnancy comes from studies of women with epilepsy rather than with bipolar disorder. These studies do show, however, that anticonvulsants rather than lithium are more closely associated with risks for birth defects. In fact, the risk of birth defects in infants born to mothers taking anticonvulsants is twice as great as that for the general population. These might include neural tube defects such as abnormal development of the spine (spina bifida) or the brain (anencephaly) as well as the atypically short nose and long upper lip known as "anticonvulsant face" that has been associated with Depakote and Tegretol specifically. Research also shows that taking two anticonvulsants in combination puts the fetus at greater risk than taking just one.

Table 2. Mood-Stabilizing Medications		
Generic name	*Trade name*	*Dose (mg/day)*
Carbamazepine	Tegretol	400–1,600
Valproic acid	Depakote (divalproex sodium)	750–2,000
Lithium carbonate	Eskalith, Lithobid, Lithonate	900–2,100
Lamotrigine	Lamictal	300–500
Gabapentin	Neurontin	900–1,800
Topiramate	Topamax	50–400

DEPAKOTE (VALPROIC ACID)

Oddly enough, Depakote was originally developed as a butter substitute in Germany during World War II, and it was not until 1963 that its anticonvulsant properties were discovered.

Now a known human teratogen, Depakote, if used during the first trimester of pregnancy, is associated with a 5 to 9 percent risk of neural tube defect. Although the risk is as high if not higher than that of Tegretol, Depakote is still more commonly used to maintain mood in bipolar patients. Like Tegretol, it is also associated with craniofacial malformations. And because the most critical time of exposure is between seventeen and thirty days after conception, most women will not know they are pregnant until after the damage is done. Preliminary findings of the Antiepileptic Drug Pregnancy Registry indicate that of 123 babies exposed, 8.9 percent were born with serious birth defects, including heart problems, so any woman taking this medication and planning a pregnancy must do whatever she can to minimize its possible effects on the fetus.

As with lithium, it is best to take Depakote in small doses throughout the day to minimize the risk of harm to the fetus. In addition, taking folic acid has been shown to reduce neural tube defects in the general population, although there is some controversy about its efficacy for women taking anticonvulsants, especially after exposure has occurred. It is recommended that women taking Depakote also take at least 4 to 5 mg of folic acid even if they are not planning a pregnancy, and those who conceive while taking the medication should begin folic acid supplementation immediately.

The effects or complications of Depakote in the newborn include withdrawal symptoms, feeding difficulties, problems with muscle tone, irritability, and jitteriness, as well as liver toxicity. Studies are currently under way to determine whether there is an increased risk of long-term neurodevelopment disorders such as autism in babies who have been exposed to this particular medication.

GUIDELINES FOR THE USE OF DEPAKOTE DURING PREGNANCY
- If you are planning a pregnancy, switch to another medication before conception if possible.

- Always take Depakote in two small doses spaced throughout the day.
- Get prenatal screening for congenital malformations. Have your serum alpha-fetoprotein levels checked to screen for neural tube defects. If these tests are positive, an amniocentesis may be indicated in order to make a full diagnosis. Fetal ultrasound at sixteen weeks is recommended.
- Take 4 to 5 mg of folic acid daily throughout the pregnancy.

TEGRETOL (CARBAMAZEPINE)

Tegretol has been associated with the craniofacial malformation known as "anticonvulsant face," as well as with a 1 percent risk of neural tube defect after first-trimester exposure. As with Depakote, therefore, women taking Tegretol should also take folic acid before and throughout their pregnancy.

Other problems linked to Tegretol include an increased risk of low birth weight, microencephaly (an abnormally small brain), and vitamin K deficiency. Because vitamin K deficiency can lead to bleeding in the fetus as well as the newborn, it is recommended that the mother take 20 mg of oral vitamin K daily during her third trimester and that the newborn receive an intramuscular injection of 1 mg vitamin K at birth. Again like Depakote, Tegretol is shown to be associated with transient liver toxicity, so the baby should be monitored.

Data on long-term neurobehavioral effects have yet to be gathered.

GUIDELINES FOR THE USE OF TEGRETOL DURING PREGNANCY

- Women taking Tegretol should be aware that it can reduce the efficacy of oral contraceptives. Women taking anticonvulsants may want to use additional precautions to prevent a pregnancy.

- Tegretol should not be administered during pregnancy unless all other options have been exhausted.

- Tegretol should not be given in combination with Depakote because the two medications taken together have a very high teratogenic effect.

- Oral supplements of 20 mg vitamin K daily throughout the third trimester and an intramuscular injection of 1 mg of vitamin K administered to the newborn at birth are recommended to reduce the risk of bleeding in the fetus and newborn.

- Women taking Tegretol should receive 4 to 5 mg of folic acid daily and should continue taking it throughout pregnancy to possibly reduce the risk of neural tube defects.

- Women who have been exposed to Tegretol at the time of conception should undergo the same prenatal testing as those taking Depakote.

LAMICTAL (LAMOTRIGINE), NEURONTIN (GABAPENTIN), AND TOPAMAX (TOPIRAMATE)

The use of Lamictal for treating bipolar women is increasing, particularly in the United States, and its manufacturer, GlaxoSmithKline, maintains a pregnancy registry that now includes almost one thousand cases. Congenital birth defects are shown to be at about 2 percent, which is equal to that of children born to unmedicated women in the general population. I would be cautious about advising my patients to take this or any of the other newer mood-stabilizing medications until we have more unbiased information and safety data available. No published data exists on Neurontin or Topamax as of this writing.

An Antiepileptic Drug Pregnancy Registry has been established and will provide more information as time goes on. The registry can be accessed by calling toll free 1-888-233-2334, or online at www. aedpregnancyregistry.org.

Treating Bipolar Disorder During Pregnancy and Postpartum

The risk factors associated with the various medications most frequently used, as well as the severity of the illness itself, can make treating bipolar disorder, particularly during pregnancy, a delicate situation for both patient and clinician.

If a prenatal screening indicates that the baby does have malformations, the mother must decide whether or not to terminate her pregnancy. For many women, however, religious, ethical, moral, or other considerations make termination out of the question, which means that they are left to deal with the almost unbearable stress of knowing that the child they are carrying may be born with one or more serious defects.

The best situation is, undoubtedly, to gradually discontinue the mood stabilizer before conception to minimize the risk of relapse as well as the risk of fetal exposure. This will also provide an opportunity for the woman to see whether or not she relapses once she is no longer taking it.

What I recommend for my own patients who want to become pregnant is that they purchase a simple ovulation kit, available at most drugstores. Then, as soon as the woman knows she is going to ovulate, she should have sexual contact. It takes two weeks from the time of conception for the connection from the uterus to the placenta (through which the medication would be transferred to the fetus) to become fully formed. During those two weeks, she can taper off her medication and then reinstate it once the first trimester is over.

Some women, of course, have no choice but to remain on medication during pregnancy, and they will require careful monitoring by a coordinated team of health care providers including their obstetrician, their psychiatrist, and a pediatrician. Through careful and skillful juggling of mood stabilizers, it is possible to ensure that the mother's illness remains in remission, that she remains stable, and that her baby is born under optimal circumstances, as was the case for Amelia, a thirty-two-year-old financial advisor who was diagnosed with bipolar illness at an early age.

She had tried a number of mood stabilizers, but the only combination that was both effective and tolerable for her was lithium (900 mg) and Depakote (500 mg). When she came to me for preconception planning, we knew our task was to keep her stable while also reducing her dosage of Depakote. In addition, we wanted to time her pregnancy so that the first trimester did not take place in winter, when many women experience an increase of depressive symptoms.

We decided to decrease the Depakote very gradually over a period of two months, and Amelia did very well for about a month after stopping the Depakote, but unfortunately she did not conceive. Within the next three months her symptoms gradually began to recur, and we had to reintroduce the Depakote.

We then waited a full year—until the following spring—at which point I first increased her dosage of lithium and then began to decrease the Depakote. This time around she did conceive while she was taking lithium alone, and once her pregnancy was confirmed, we reduced the Lithium from 1,200 mg to 900 and then to 600 throughout the first trimester.

At sixteen weeks Amelia went for an ultrasound, which ruled out Ebstein's anomaly. Even though she was not taking Depakote, because she was in her mid-thirties at the time we also did an alpha-fetoprotein test to rule out Down syndrome and other malformations.

Her pregnancy proceeded absolutely normally, and in the third trimester we began to test her lithium levels regularly to be sure they remained at a therapeutic level. When we noticed that the level had decreased near the end of her pregnancy, we debated whether or not to increase the dose. But because she remained symptom free, we decided simply to monitor her closely. During labor, we kept her on 600 mg rather than reducing the dose any further.

Amelia gave birth to a healthy baby and immediately increased her lithium to 900 mg. A week later we also reintroduced her Depakote, and she chose not to breast-feed in order to avoid the risk of exposing her newborn to the medication. By two weeks after giving birth she was back on her preconception levels of lithium and Depakote, and now, two years later, both Amelia and her baby are doing very well.

The point of Amelia's story is to indicate that even if a woman has bipolar disorder, she can conceive and successfully carry a healthy baby to term without endangering her own health. But the pregnancy needs to be carefully planned and monitored.

Pregnancy does appear to be protective of bipolar symptoms for a small number of women who have experienced only one bipolar episode. These women are able to discontinue their medication during pregnancy without relapsing, although they still run the risk of relapsing postpartum. For most, however, this is not the case, and it's impossible to know in advance which way it will go. With that in mind, taking a let's-see-what-happens approach to conception would be irresponsible for both the woman and her physician.

Typical and Atypical Antipsychotics

With the advent of antipsychotics at the beginning of the twentieth century, thousands of institutionalized mental patients were "miraculously cured." Thorazine (chlorpromazine), the first of the antipsychotics, was developed by a French surgeon, Dr. Henri Laborit, for use as an anesthetic. As is the case with so many psychotropic medications, its calming and antipsychotic properties were discovered only later. The newer (so-called novel or atypical) antipsychotics, however, have been developed with the more recent and sophisticated knowledge we now have about the way particular neurotransmitters—in this case dopamine specifically—affect the function of the brain.

Table 3. CLASSIFICATIONS OF ANTIPSYCHOTIC MEDICATIONS					
Conventional (Typical) Antipsychotics			**Novel (Atypical) Antipsychotics**		
Generic name	*Trade name*	*Dose (mg/day)*	*Generic name*	*Trade name*	*Dose (mg/day)*
Haloperidol	Haldol	5–10	Clozapine	Clozaril	100–450
Pimozide	Orap	1–10	Risperidone	Risperdal	1–6
Chlorpromazine	Thorazine Largactil	200–800	Olanzapine	Zyprexa	5–20
Fluphenazine	Perimitil Prolixin	5–10	Quetiapine	Seroquel	25–600
Perphenazine	Trilafon	8–32			
Thioridazine	Melleril	200–600			
Trifluoperazine	Stelazine	10–40			

THE RISKS AND BENEFITS OF CONVENTIONAL (TYPICAL) ANTIPSYCHOTICS

The bulk of our information about the adverse effects of conventional antipsychotics comes from their use by pregnant women who were not necessarily psychotic but who were being studied because they were suffering from hyperemesis gravidarum, or excessive vomiting. In a large study of 75,000 live births at least 2,500 of the participants had been exposed to phenothiazines, a group of conventional antipsychotics, during their first trimester. The study found that the relative risk of malformation was approximately 0.4 percent (4 in 1,000), higher than the normal baseline risk of 1 to 2 percent, and also that the low-potency antipsychotics such as Thorazine were more teratogenic than the high-potency typical antipsychotics such as Haldol.

It should be noted, however, that many researchers now believe that the untreated disease may, in and of itself, be responsible for increasing the risk of fetal malformation. Further, women who are psychotic may engage in behaviors such as substance abuse and poor prenatal care that could also account for some increased malformation. Many psychiatrists are, in fact, more comfortable prescribing the older antipsychotics than they are with the newer ones because there is more available data about them.

Both Haldol and Thorazine have been associated with infant withdrawal symptoms including tremors, restlessness, and feeding difficulties, but most of these symptoms resolve within a few days, and some researchers believe that they result from the mother's taking additional medications that are sometimes needed to counteract the side effects of the antipsychotics.

Studies of children up to five years of age have shown no long-term effects on intellectual functioning of their exposure to the typical antipsychotics, and although these drugs do have many side effects (including those mentioned above), they continue to have a place in the treatment of psychotic illness during pregnancy.

THE RISKS AND BENEFITS OF NOVEL (ATYPICAL) ANTIPSYCHOTICS

Information about the reproductive safety of the newer anti-psychotics is still very limited. The older antipsychotics were known to cause infertility, and some of the newer ones may affect fertility as well. But others, most notably Seroquel (quetiapine), do not have this effect. These medications are now the treatment of choice for both bipolar illness and schizophrenia. Many patients are not able to tolerate the side effects of the older antipsychotics, and the advent of these atypical antipsychotics has had a significant impact on the way psychotic illness is managed today.

Many clinicians believe they are safer to use as mood stabilizers during pregnancy than the anticonvulsants, which, as I've discussed, are known to be teratogenic. Therefore, many women who discontinue their anticonvulsants during pregnancy have benefited from taking atypical antipsychotics to control their symptoms.

Barbi, who had a ten-year history of bipolar disorder, had been stabilized on 750 mg of Depakote daily. A social worker at a large cancer institute, Barbi had seen a lot of sadness in her professional life and was not prepared to deal with the personal sadness of giving birth to a baby with spina bifida or some other serious defect.

When she came to me for a preconception consultation, we ultimately decided, after much discussion of the risks and benefits, to wean her off the Depakote and start her on 1 mg of Risperdal (risperidone). Happily, she conceived, remained asymptomatic throughout her pregnancy, and delivered a healthy baby.

After giving birth, Barbi decided to breast-feed her baby while taking the Risperdal. During that time we collected her breast milk to measure the levels of medication for a study we are currently undertaking to determine how antipsychotic medications are transferred through breast milk. After six weeks, she stopped nursing and began to taper off the Risperdal and reintroduce the Depakote.

Switching a patient from an anticonvulsant to an antipsychotic medication is complicated, requires careful handling, and is not something that is commonly undertaken at this time. More research must be done before we determine how effective or risky this method of treatment can be. It is, however, an alternative that may work for a number of patients, and one that any woman who does not want to take Depakote or another anticonvulsant during pregnancy should consider in consultation with her physician.

Clozaril (clozapine)

One of the first atypical antipsychotics, Clozaril is not known to cause any major congenital malformations. The original registry established by its manufacturer now includes twenty-eight cases, twenty-five of which were healthy births, while the remaining three each had a different birth defect. Among adults taking Clozaril, however, about 1 percent experience a deficiency of white blood cells, so infants who have been exposed require testing to determine their white blood cell count. If there is a problem, discontinue the medication and the condition will resolve itself.

Risperdal (risperidone)

To date, there are only two case reports of Risperdal use throughout pregnancy, but in both instances the babies were delivered at term by elective cesarean section with no neonatal or maternal complications. Both babies were then followed up to twelve months of age and showed no developmental abnormalities. But with only two cases to go by, it's much too early to make any kind of general recommendation about the risk/benefit ratio of this medication.

Zyprexa (olanzapine)

The manufacturer's safety database for Zyprexa includes data on a total of ninety-six exposed infants with only one report of a major malformation. The risks for women using Zyprexa during pregnancy include increased weight gain, gestational diabetes, and preeclampsia, so these women should be sure that their weight, blood sugar levels, and blood pressure are carefully monitored.

Seroquel (quetiapine)

Quetiapine is being used increasingly to control mania and to stabilize mood. The current data include only two cases with no reports of perinatal complications. In our clinic we are using this medication with increasing frequency because of its calming and sedating properties and less extrapyramidal side effects.

GUIDELINES FOR THE USE OF ATYPICAL ANTIPSYCHOTICS DURING PREGNANCY

- If a woman becomes pregnant while taking an atypical antipsychotic, she may have to continue taking it in order to avoid the risk of relapse while changing medications.

- If a woman relapses during pregnancy while off the medication or develops a new psychotic illness during pregnancy, it is best to put her on an antipsychotic to which she has responded well in the past. If possible, in my own opinion, an atypical antipsychotic would be the best choice because they have fewer side effects than the older medications, which means that the patient will be more likely to comply with the treatment.

- In every case, the risk of taking the medication must be weighed against the risk of allowing the psychosis to go untreated.

Because antipsychotic medications are very strong, we normally prescribe them only for those women who are delusional, have experienced hallucinations, or have obsessional thoughts so severe that they may border on becoming psychotic. In some cases, such as that of my patient Anka, however, they are indicated and can be extremely effective. Anka had come to Canada from a war-ravaged country; as a result of her environment, she had grown up feeling extremely unsafe and suspicious. She had learned early on to be careful, to always look over her shoulder, and not to trust anyone. In other words, being suspicious was a normal part of her personality.

When Anka became pregnant, she began to have thoughts of her baby being taken away from her and made to fight in the ongoing war. Even though she recognized how ludicrous and ridiculous these thoughts really were, they became more frequent and vivid as her pregnancy progressed until they became a fixed, full-blown delusion without any symptoms of depression. Unusual as this may be, such a delusion can and did happen.

To resolve her paranoid thinking we started Anka on 50 mg of Seroquel twice daily, increasing the dose to 200 and then 300 mg, at which point she finally responded. Her pregnancy progressed with no further problems after that, and we continued the medication throughout her second and third trimesters and for the first three months postpartum, after which we began to gradually wean her from the drug. As we continued to monitor her closely, it became apparent that she was beginning to show symptoms of bipolar disorder, so eventually we put her on a mood stabilizer in addition to the Seroquel, and she has remained stable since that time.

Benzodiazepines

In the early 1900s phenobarbital was introduced as the first sleeping pill. Although it was used mainly to control seizures in patients with epilepsy, it worked as a sedative and also had anxiety-reducing properties. Its anticonvulsant properties caused researchers to synthesize nonsedative anticonvulsants, which led eventually to the development of the first benzodiazepine, Librium (chlordiazepoxide).

Although benzodiazepines are much safer than barbitals, they are also highly addictive; as a result, many people tend to abuse them and become dependent on them. They are, however, commonly prescribed for anxiety disorders and sleep disorders. They are used as antiepileptic medications, and they have muscle-relaxant properties.

Given their drawbacks, one might wonder why they would ever be prescribed during pregnancy, but a Swedish study headed by Dr. Ulf Bergman that looked at prescribing practices in the United States found that 2 percent of women who were receiving Medicaid benefits filled one or more prescriptions for benzodiazepines during pregnancy. Since many pregnancies are, as I've already stated, unplanned, women may easily be taking these medications and expose their fetus during the first trimester without realizing it. Beyond concerns of early exposure, however, there is the further concern about the withdrawal effects on the newborn of benzodiazepines taken during the third trimester.

In general, these medications are prescribed to control generalized anxiety disorder, obsessive-compulsive disorder, or panic disorder in pregnancy. They are also used to control sleep deprivation in patients with bipolar disorder, and in combination with an SSRI for those who are depressed and anxious.

They are also useful for controlling or alleviating medical disorders associated with pregnancy, including eclampsia or preeclampsia, anxiety associated with third-trimester placental bleeding, and preterm labor. They may also be used as a light anesthetic when needed to perform a procedure during pregnancy, at induction of labor, or before a C-section.

The stories of two of my patients illustrate how short-term use of benzodiazepines during pregnancy can result in positive outcomes.

Adele, at twenty-eight weeks gestation, woke up in the middle of the night experiencing acute pain, severe cramping, and bleeding. Frightened to death, she thought she was going into labor and awakened her husband in a state of frenzy. She arrived at my hospital by ambulance and was given 2 mg of Ativan to calm her down. As the cramping and bleeding continued, her anxiety became so acute that the obstetrician overseeing her case called our clinic, where I happened to be on call.

When I saw Adele, I prescribed 2 mg of Ativan daily for the next five days, during which time the bleeding stopped, her anxiety levels dropped, and she was gradually weaned from the Ativan. After being put on bed rest, she gave birth to a full-term, healthy baby girl.

In another acute situation, Aurelia's water broke in the middle of the night (when it seems so many complications occur) when she was twenty-nine weeks pregnant, and she, like Adele, arrived at the hospital by ambulance. She was given 2 mg of Klonopin immediately, and the medication was continued at 1 to 2 mg daily as needed for the next week, until the leaking from her membranes finally stopped. The Klonopin helped to calm the anxiety associated with her possibly going into early labor, and eventually she delivered at full term.

In situations like these, not using benzodiazepines could have led to more complications caused by the situation itself than those potentially caused by the medication.

THE RISKS AND BENEFITS OF USING BENZODIAZEPINES

Benzodiazepines are categorized into four groups, according to their half-life—the length of time it takes the body to clear half the drug from the system, which is a reflection of how long the drug itself will have an effect. The four groups are:

1. Those with a half-life of forty-eight hours or more. Valium (diazepam) and Librium (chlordiazepoxide) belong to this group.
2. Those with a half-life of twenty-four to forty-eight hours. Klonopin (clonazepam) belongs to this group.
3. Those with a half-life of ten to twenty-four hours. Ativan (lorazepam) belongs to this group.
4. Those with a half-life of ten hours or less. Xanax (alprazolam) belongs to this group.

The table below shows the FDA categories for the various benzodiazepines.

Table 4. CLASSIFICATIONS OF BENZODIAZEPINES

Generic name	Trade name	FDA pregnancy category	Suggested daily dosage range (mg)
Clonazepam	Klonopin	C	0.5–4
Lorazepam	Ativan	D	2–6
Alprazolam	Xanax	D	0.5–6.0
Diazepam	Valium	D	2–60
Chlordiazepoxide	Libritabs Librium	D	15–100

A brilliant review conducted by members of the pharmacology department of the Motherisk Program looked at fourteen hundred studies, including twenty-three that examined the use of benzodiazepines during pregnancy, in order to determine the frequency of malformations, particularly the incidence of cleft palate and/or cleft lip associated with first-trimester exposure. The researchers found an association between benzodiazepines and cleft palate in a small percentage of cases, but they cautioned that this finding was not completely reliable because of inconsistencies in the original research. So even in a worst-case scenario benzodiazepines do not appear to be significant human teratogens.

The fear that was associated with use of the older benzodiazepines does not appear to be substantiated with the newer, shorter-acting medications that are now most commonly prescribed during pregnancy. In the review that follows—going from the shortest- to the longest-acting—I will look at Xanax, Ativan, and Klonopin, the three that are used most frequently, and, for purposes of historical perspective and comparison, Valium.

Xanax (alprazolam)

Several studies of women exposed to Xanax during the first trimester show no association with congenital malformation. There are, however, reports of transient neonatal withdrawal symptoms, especially when Xanax is given during late pregnancy, that include tremors, poor muscle tone, and respiratory difficulty. One of the main problems associated with Xanax is that because it has such a short half-life, many women taking it experience a "rebound phenomenon," meaning that as soon as it wears off, they need to take more immediately. For that reason, I tend to avoid using it in my own clinical practice.

Ativan (lorazepam)

Although human reproductive data is quite limited, Ativan is not considered to be teratogenic in animals. There have been some case reports that associate its use with a variety of malformations, but one study of women taking Ativan during pregnancy, although the sample size was small, did not show any increase in the pattern of malformation, especially when exposure occurred during the first trimester.

Because it is often used near the onset of labor, exposure may occasionally cause transient neonatal respiratory distress, lower scores on Apgar tests (performed to assess the newborn's condition based on activity, pulse, grimace, appearance, and respiration at one and five minutes after birth), and feeding problems, but none of these has been shown to have any long-term consequences.

Klonopin (clonazepam)

Despite the occasional case report of malformation associated with Klonopin, studies have shown no consistent causality related to exposure during pregnancy. Dr. Lisa Weinstock of Massachusetts General Hospital, in association with Dr. Lee Cohen, conducted a study of thirty-eight women with panic disorder who had taken Klonopin during pregnancy and found that it produced few problems associated either with malformation or with neonatal withdrawal. And a study we recently completed at my own hospital found no babies exposed to Klonopin in the first trimester who were born with any abnormalities or malformations.

We, along with other researchers at my hospital, however, have found that third-trimester exposure may be associated with symptoms of neonatal withdrawal, which are, as I've said, short-lived and easily resolved. In our own clinic, we prescribe Klonopin far more often than any other benzodiazepine because it is neither as short-lived as Xanax nor as long-lasting as Valium.

Valium (diazepam)

Until the early 1980s Valium was the most frequently prescribed benzodiazepine in the United States. At present, however, its use is generally limited to treating acute withdrawal from alcohol, other long-acting benzodiazepines, or barbiturates; in conjunction with anticonvulsant medications; and occasionally as a light preoperative anesthetic.

Several early case-controlled studies found it to be associated with a significantly increased risk of oral cleft, but the current understanding among clinicians is that the risk is unlikely. That said, however, in my clinic we rarely prescribe Valium, which can remain in the body for up to one hundred hours, preferring to use one of the newer, shorter-acting medications now available.

GUIDELINES FOR THE USE OF BENZODIAZEPINES
DURING PREGNANCY

- It would be prudent to avoid the use of benzodiazepines during the first trimester unless they are absolutely necessary for symptom relief. If using one of these medications is indicated, it would be best to stick with either Klonopin or Ativan, neither of which has been associated with fetal malformation.

- During the third trimester, to reduce the risk of neonatal withdrawal, restrict the use of benzodiazepines in combination with other medications.

- Always use the lowest effective dose for the shortest possible time, and only when the patient is symptomatic.

- Smaller, more frequent doses are recommended to avoid concentrations peaking and falling.

- Be aware of the risk for dependency even after use for a relatively short period of time. Exposure should be limited to no more than two weeks.

- Any concern about the risk for oral cleft can be resolved with a level-two ultrasound to visualize the defect early in pregnancy. But, as I have said, the risk of this particular malformation is unlikely, particularly with the newer benzodiazepines.

- Lastly, if symptoms return after discontinuing benzodiazepines, then continue their use cautiously.

Electroconvulsive Therapy

As far back as the 1930s camphor-induced seizures were used as a means of treating the severely mentally ill. In 1938 Drs. Ugo Cerletti and Lucio Bini first used electric current to control delusions and hallucinations in a schizophrenic male.

To this day, however, the media continue to depict electroconvulsive therapy (ECT) in a horrific and distorted way. Simply mentioning ECT immediately conjures up images of terrifying scenes from *One Flew Over the Cuckoo's Nest* and *A Beautiful Mind*. But ECT plays an important role in the treatment of psychiatric illness, and these movie scenes bear no resemblance to the reality of how it is administered today in a hospital setting.

The American Psychiatric Association has very specific guidelines for the use of electroconvulsive therapy:

- It is to be used only to treat severe, debilitating mental disorders after other therapies have failed and/or medication has not proved effective.
- It is to be considered only when there is imminent risk of suicide that requires quicker results than can be obtained through the use of medication.
- It requires the patient's informed consent.

Brianna's case indicates how, in the rare but critical situation, ECT can be a lifesaving procedure.

Brianna was eight weeks into an unplanned pregnancy when she became psychotic, with delusions that her food was being poisoned. In fact, she was so convinced that her food and water were being contaminated that she was literally starving at the point when I received an urgent call from her family doctor.

Although Brianna denied any prior history of mental illness, it became clear when I talked to her family that she had barely recovered from a previous untreated depressive episode when she became pregnant. Already the mother of four, she was extremely thin and frail, weighing only about ninety pounds, and was also acutely suicidal.

Had we not intervened and immediately administered ECT, it is probable that she would have died. Instead, after eight treatments she showed a dramatic improvement and gave birth to a healthy baby.

Electroconvulsive therapy works by temporarily altering the electrochemical processes in the brain. It does not, as some apparently believe, cause premature labor or contraction of the uterine muscle during seizure. As it is administered today, for patients with no other choice, it is quite safe, with a mortality rate of 1 in 1,000—and those deaths are often due to the use of anesthetic rather than to the actual procedure.

No matter how you look at it, the treatment isn't pleasant. The patient is anesthetized and receives electrical impulses that change brain chemistry. She wakes up confused, and the memory loss can be very frightening. But having used ECT on many patients both during pregnancy and postpartum, and having seen them recover dramatically without prolonged suffering, I can say with confidence that in those cases it was the correct choice of treatment.

To provide another case history, this one of a woman who received ECT postpartum, I would like to share the story of Peggy, who was admitted to the psychiatric ward of our hospital.

Peggy had been adopted as an infant, and while she loved her adoptive parents, she began to search for her biological mother as soon as she was of age to do so. When she found her, however, Peggy's birth mother was reluctant to connect with her. As it turned out, she'd given birth to Peggy when she was just eighteen years old and had had a psychotic breakdown that required hospitalization shortly thereafter. Having given Peggy up, she wanted to erase all those bad memories, including her daughter.

Subsequently, feeling disillusioned as well as once more abandoned and rejected, Peggy began to believe that since her mother had rejected her, she in turn might reject her own child if she had one. It took many months of psychotherapy before she was able to grasp the fact that her own circumstances were different from her mother's and feel that she was ready to have a baby.

Peggy's husband had lost his father at a very young age and deeply longed to make up for that loss by being a good father himself. So when Peggy finally did become pregnant, both she and her husband felt that they were absolutely prepared for parenthood. Her pregnancy was a breeze, and when she gave birth to her daughter, Alicia, both she and her husband took parental leave, vowing that they would be "perfect parents" and that neither of them would ever abandon their child as they had been abandoned.

Shortly after coming home from the hospital, however, Peggy began to have unusual feelings of hostility toward her baby. At first she couldn't understand where her feelings of anger were coming from. Her husband noticed that Peggy would let Alicia cry for hours in her crib without going to comfort her. But when he questioned her behavior, Peggy told him she'd read a book that said if she "spoiled" the baby too much by taking her from the crib, she would become too dependent on her mother. Since this was the first experience of parenting for both of them, Peggy's husband didn't argue with her until he began to realize that her behavior toward Alicia was actually bordering on neglect.

When I saw Peggy in my office, she was delusional. She believed the baby was a monster and was telling her that she was a bad person. Every time Alicia cried, Peggy had thoughts of wanting to harm her. When he heard her telling me these things, Peggy's husband broke down and cried. It was clear that she was extremely ill and needed immediate help. Her baby was now four months old, and her delusions were getting worse as time went on.

Because she was considered to be a risk to herself and others and was not capable of giving informed consent, she was admitted to the hospital involuntarily with her husband's consent and received ECT. After the fourth treatment, she began to improve dramatically, to the point where she was able to hold her baby. Every day Peggy's aunt brought Alicia to the hospital, and Peggy began to connect with her for the first time. Although her short-term memory was temporarily affected because of the treatment, her confusion and memory loss disappeared after a few months and she was able to establish a normal, loving relationship with her daughter.

Leaving a woman in Peggy's condition to care for a baby would have been, in my opinion, unethical, improper, and inhumane. My experience with the effectiveness of ECT in her case and the cases of other women in similarly critical states has taught me that, when used properly, it is a safe and effective treatment for some patients who are severely distressed and disturbed.

A Word to the Burdened but Brave

Any woman who is emotionally ill carries a tremendous burden. Those who are willing to accept and seek treatment for their illness while at the same time retaining their desire for and devotion to motherhood are, to my mind, supremely courageous. I am amazed on a daily basis by their resolve to overcome any obstacle in order to become a healthy, responsible, and loving parent, and because of that, I am constantly renewed in my own resolve to bring their problems to greater attention and help them in whatever way I can.

9

Breast-feeding and Medication

THE RISKS AND THE BENEFITS

The American Academy of Pediatrics endorses breast-feeding as the best source of nutrition for infants in the first six months of life. The World Health Organization promotes its benefits globally. Private organizations advocate it with mailings sent to new mothers. Women are told by friends, family, and a significant portion of society that if they don't breast-feed, they are somehow less good mothers than those who do.

Historically, attitudes toward breast-feeding have varied from century to century and country to country. In some societies *not* to breast-feed is considered a mark of sophistication. In others, breast-feeding is a way of life. And in some ancient cultures wet nurses were hired specifically to nurse other women's new babies. In modern Western culture, however, at least for the past twenty years, it has become abundantly clear that breast-feeding is considered synonymous with motherhood. Breast milk is healthy from a nutritional point of view; it is believed to protect the baby from certain illnesses; it's cheap; and in most cases it's readily available. In addition, it gives mothers the opportunity to nurture, bond with, and express feelings of love for their newborn in a very special way.

The decision to breast-feed is not, however, always so simple, especially for women who suffer from depression and are taking psychotropic medications.

Postpartum Depression

In the United States there are approximately four million babies born every year, and nearly half of all new mothers will breast-feed their infants. Since postpartum depression affects between 10 and 13 percent of all women, it can be assumed that some new mothers will be nursing while they are taking antidepressants.

The differences between postpartum blues, postpartum depression, and psychosis are for the most part a matter of duration and degree. Postpartum blues are characterized by increased emotionality, fluctuating moods, crying spells, anxiety related to the newborn, and increased irritability. These symptoms, however, are generally quite transitory and resolve themselves within a week or two. They peak approximately three to five days after delivery, during which time the mother may require support, reassurance, and occasionally medication to help her sleep.

Approximately one in ten of all new mothers will, however, develop full-blown postpartum depression. This is particularly true of women who have a personal or family history of depression or who have experienced a previous postpartum depression. Many of these will be happily married, will have had a perfectly happy pregnancy, and will have delivered a healthy baby with no complications.

Although the *DSM-IV-TR* defines a major depression as "postpartum" only if its onset occurs during the first four weeks after childbirth, researchers and clinicians working in the area of reproductive psychiatry understand that the postpartum period extends at least up to six months and that postpartum depression can manifest itself for up to a year after childbirth, particularly if the mother is breast-feeding. Some women nurse their babies for six to eight months, during which time they *may* be protected from depression by the continued production of prolactin, the nursing hormone. If this is the case—and it is certainly *not* the case for *all* women—depression may not make itself known until after they stop breast-feeding.

Mental illness associated with childbirth was first documented by Hippocrates in 400 BCE; it was also noted by Trotula, a female doctor in Salerno, Italy, in her eleventh-century work, *The Diseases of Women*. In 1858 Dr. Jean Etienne Esquirol, a well-known French psychiatrist, also made a connection between lactation and mental illness in women. Yet even today we are still struggling to understand how best to treat postpartum depression without causing harm to either mother or baby. One of the most serious questions related to treating the illness involves the dilemma women face when deciding whether or not to breast-feed while taking antidepressant medication or, conversely, whether or not to take antidepressants while breast-feeding.

The Questions Every Nursing Mother Asks

Invariably, a woman will ask questions when her doctor diagnoses her depression because the next decision she has to make, if the doctor feels she needs medication, is a difficult one, both for her and her caregiver.

1. Am I really depressed? Is the diagnosis of depression a correct one?
2. Can I get better without the antidepressants?
3. Should I try other forms of therapy before I resort to taking drugs while I'm nursing?
4. If I must take these drugs, what does my doctor know about them?
5. How much of this drug is secreted in my breast milk?
6. How much of this drug will my baby be exposed to?
7. Will my baby be affected in any way if I nurse while taking these drugs?
8. What will be the short- and long-term effects on my baby?

Starting out, I have to say that I don't like to use the term *drugs*, which to me carries a negative connotation associated with illicit substances.

In fact, one concern I always have when depression goes untreated is that women will turn to substances such as cigarettes, alcohol, or marijuana in order to self-medicate and alleviate the pain they are feeling.

As with antenatal depression, decisions about how and when to treat postpartum depression can only be made by a patient in consultation with her doctor. Put as simply as possible, there are really three choices:

1. Expose the baby to medication through the breast milk.
2. Expose the baby to the adverse effects of untreated depression in the mother.
3. Take antidepressant medications and don't breast-feed the baby.

How to Minimize Your Baby's Exposure

The first thing to understand is that the composition of breast milk varies according to when the milk is produced. The first milk produced in the earliest days of breast-feeding is called colostrum. It's low in fat and high in carbohydrates and protein as well as in the antibodies that help to keep your baby healthy. It's unclear at this time whether or not medications pass through the colostrum, since the milk is immature at this point and does not reach its stable composition for about two weeks.

The first part of the milk the baby sucks during a feeding is called foremilk, and the last is called hindmilk. Medications—particularly some of the SSRIs such as Zoloft—appear to be more concentrated in the hindmilk, which is richer in fat content than the foremilk.

Levels of various medication peak in the breast milk at different times. Some, including Zoloft, peak eight to nine hours after they are taken. This is significant because if she knows when the level of the medication peaks, the nursing mother can minimize her baby's exposure by about 20 percent if she pumps and discards the milk that is produced at the time of greatest concentration. Or she can nurse and then take the medication immediately after.

And finally, which medication she takes can also make a significant difference. In a pooled analysis of the available data from fifty-seven studies on antidepressant levels in nursing infants, recently published in the *American Journal of Psychiatry,* Dr. Alicia Weissman and her colleagues from the University of Iowa conclude that among the SSRIs, Paxil and Zoloft may be the preferred choices for breast-feeding women because of their almost undetectable levels when measured in the infant's blood. They also noted that of drugs commonly used, Prozac produces the highest infant levels. Similar findings were replicated by my colleagues and me with respect to Paxil, Zoloft, and Prozac. We are presently researching the levels of Celexa and Effexor in breast milk and the baby's blood.

At present we are studying other factors that may affect the baby's level of exposure, including the pH level of the milk and maternal blood as well as particular characteristics of the medication itself, such as its half-life, its molecular weight, and the presence or absence of breakdown products.

Monitoring the Baby's Exposure

At this time, there have been no systematic, long-term follow-up studies of babies who were exposed to medications through their mother's breast milk. Currently, our research group at British Columbia Women's Hospital is conducting such a study by assessing the neurological development of children exposed to Paxil, Effexor, and Celexa, but so far, most of the information we have is anecdotal in nature. The good news, however, is that research to date indicates that the levels of medication transferred to the infant are far lower than those in the mother's blood and in some cases are actually undetectable.

Currently, the preferred method of monitoring infant exposure is to measure the level of medication in the infant's blood where this service is possible. Unfortunately, however, this kind of testing is not always available, and many laboratories do not have equipment sensitive enough to obtain accurate results. The older, more common way of testing is to measure the amount of medication in the mother's blood and the amount found in her breast milk, and approximate the exposure depending on the infant's weight.

Perhaps the best way to determine how a baby is being affected by medication, however, is for the mother to be attentive and alert to how her child is behaving. Does the baby seem too drowsy, irritable, or fussy? If so, the mother needs to discuss these symptoms with her doctor. Most mothers are exquisitely aware of any small change in their infant, and anyone who feels that her baby is being adversely affected by her medication may decide to either try a lower dose or stop breast-feeding. It is critical, however, that she *not* abruptly discontinue her medication because her risk of relapse would then be extremely high.

Randi was not uncomfortable with the idea of breast-feeding her baby while taking Wellbutrin, as she had responded to Wellbutrin earlier. She'd experienced postpartum depression after the birth of her first child and remembered nursing mechanically without ever feeling any connection with her infant, so she wanted to do things differently the second time around. This time she wanted to enjoy the experience and feel the love and attachment she'd so desperately missed.

We started her on a daily dose of 100 mg of Wellbutrin SR, increased it to 200 mg the following week, and then raised it to 300 mg after four weeks. At that dose, however, Randi noticed that her baby was not sleeping, had become more irritable, and was fussing a lot more than usual. We recommended that she stop taking the Wellbutrin and begin taking Paxil CR instead. We explained that we would gradually wean her from the Wellbutrin and introduce a small dose of the Paxil CR, which we would slowly increase to a therapeutic level. Randi, however, decided that she did not want to continue nursing if doing so meant that she would be exposing her baby to two medications.

Maggie's story is somewhat different. She was experiencing her first episode of postpartum depression and was taking Paxil. After discussing the risks and benefits of nursing while taking the medication, and even though the information we have about Paxil is quite positive (the levels found in breast milk are generally undetectable), she decided not to breast-feed. The decision wasn't easy for her; she thought about it for a long time. Ultimately, however, she chose to err on the side of caution.

Clearly, what is the right decision for one woman will not be right for another.

Antidepressants and Breast-feeding: Which Ones Are Best?

Selective Serotonin Reuptake Inhibitors (SSRIs)

Because SSRIs are now commonly used for nursing mothers, we have gathered more data on them than on any of the other psychotropic medications currently in use. With time, more data on Effexor will be available. I have compiled the following chart, based on published studies, to show the adverse outcomes for infants whose mothers took various SSRIs.

Medication	Number of babies in whom medication blood levels were measured	Adverse events in the infant reported
Prozac (fluoxetine)	79	3—colic, gastric upset 1—irritability 1—unresponsiveness 4—high infant serum
Zoloft (sertraline)	108	None reported in 106 infants 2—high infant serum
Paxil (paroxetine)	66	None reported in any infants
Effexor (venlafaxine)	12	None reported in any infants
Celexa (citalopram)	18	None reported in 17 infants 1—uneasy sleep
Wellbutrin (bupropion)	3	None reported in any infants

At this time seventy-nine infants exposed to Prozac have been studied. One of the larger studies, which compared twenty-six Prozac-treated mother-infant pairs to thirty-eight controls, found that those infants who had been exposed weighed slightly less than those in the control group. Of the total ninety-two on whom we have data, however, only five have shown minor behavioral symptoms such as colic and hyperactivity, while the vast majority do not show any adverse outcomes at all.

Results of the research on seventy-seven babies exposed to Paxil and 146 exposed to Zoloft have also been positive, with infant medication levels that are almost undetectable.

This is important information both for the prescribing doctor and for the patient since Paxil and Zoloft are also the two SSRIs shown to be effective in the treatment of postpartum depression. Dr. Kathy Wisner and her group from Case Western Reserve University in Cleveland recently published a study in the *American Journal of Psychiatry* reporting the suppression of postpartum symptoms with Zoloft (sertraline). And my own study published in the September 2004 issue of the *Clinical Journal of Psychiatry* describes the effectiveness of Paxil in the treatment of postpartum depression in nursing mothers.

We are still collecting more information on milk levels of Effexor, although its efficacy in treatment of postpartum depression has been demonstrated. With Celexa and Wellbutrin, at the moment there have been no reported problems other than transient and reversible sleep difficulties shown in one infant exposed to Celexa. Minimizing the maternal dose of Celexa may be helpful. No data at all are currently available on infant exposure to Remeron.

Tricyclic Antidepressants and Monoamine Oxidase Inhibitors (MAOIs)

Although they are as effective as SSRIs, tricyclic antidepressants are no longer commonly prescribed for depression because of their many side effects, which include weight gain, sedation, and lowering blood pressure, as well as the risk of taking a fatal overdose.

They are, however, quite safe for breast-feeding mothers, although clinicians generally recommend nortriptyline or desipramine, both of which have the fewest side effects.

MAOIs are also used infrequently because of the dietary restrictions they require and their tendency to spike blood pressure. They are not recommended for use by nursing mothers.

Mood Stabilizers and Breast-feeding

Lithium

The American Academy of Pediatrics recommends caution for women who are breast-feeding while taking lithium, as some studies have found lithium levels in the infant blood to be as high as one-half to one-third of the therapeutic levels in the maternal blood. The excretion of lithium into the breast milk is higher than for any other psychotropic medicine I have described thus far. In our own clinic, we generally advise women not to breast-feed while taking lithium, but if they insist on nursing, we monitor the baby's lithium levels very closely and advise them to keep the infant well hydrated with plenty of fluids to avoid excess accumulation of the medicine, which could lead to toxicity. In a recent publication, Dr. Kim Yonkers of Yale University, along with a group of experts, recommended that lithium-exposed infants should have regular blood tests.

Depakote (valproic acid)

The American Academy of Pediatrics has designated Depakote "compatible with breast-feeding." It is excreted into the breast milk in small amounts and appears to be safe. Infants should, however, be monitored for liver function because some cases of toxic effects on the liver have been reported. In one documented report, a three-month-old developed a low level of blood platelets (thrombocytopenia) and anemia, but these abnormalities were resolved when breast-feeding was stopped. Many clinicians recommend not nursing while on Depakote.

Tegretol (carbamazepine)

Both Tegretol and its major metabolites are excreted in the breast milk, and although the amount of transfer is quite low, it's important to measure the baby's liver enzymes, as there have been two reported incidents of liver toxicity in babies exposed to Tegretol. In one case, however, the mother was taking the medication both during pregnancy and post-partum, so it's difficult to determine whether the toxicity was caused from the baby's exposure in utero or through the breast milk. The message here is that if you must breast-feed while taking this (or any) medication, make sure your baby is closely monitored.

Lamictal (lamotrigine), Neurontin (gabapentin), and Topamax (topiramate)

Although there is some concern about skin rashes, information available on the use of Lamictal while breast-feeding is extremely limited, and the American Academy of Pediatrics has classified it "unknown but may be of concern."

We have no data at all on either Neurontin or Topamax.

Antipsychotics

We have information on twenty-eight infants exposed to typical or older antipsychotics through nursing, and in the majority of cases no adverse events or side effects have been reported.

Of the newer or atypical antipsychotics, there have been fifteen reports of infants exposed to Zyprexa through lactation, one of whom was found to have jaundice, lethargy, and a heart murmur. Three case reports detailing a total of six exposures to Risperdal found no significant hazard in the short term. Finally, the information on Seroquel is still virtually nonexistent, but we are collecting samples at my own clinic, and results of our analyses will be available shortly.

Benzodiazepines

Although they do not have any known adverse effects on the infant, benzodiazepines are not considered ideal for use during breast-feeding, both because of their relatively long half-lives and because of the risk for dependency. If they are prescribed, it would be best to use those that are intermediate-acting (Ativan or Klonopin), which are eliminated relatively quickly from the mother, and only for a short period of time. Withdrawal symptoms have been reported in one infant exposed to Xanax through breast-feeding. Of fourteen reported cases in which infants were exposed to Klonopin, there was one report of transitory respiratory difficulty, but the problem was quickly resolved. No adverse effects have been reported with relation to Ativan.

GUIDELINES FOR THE USE OF MEDICATIONS WHILE BREAST-FEEDING

1. Maternal factors
   a. Accurate diagnosis of the postpartum psychiatric condition is important.
   b. Nonpharmacological, alternative therapies should first be explored in cases of mild to moderate illness.
2. Medication factors
   a. Make sure that the medicine has some proven safety record during breast-feeding.
   b. Make sure that you try to use agents that do not readily pass into the breast milk.
   c. Use the lowest possible dose necessary to achieve symptom remission.
   d. Choose a medication that has no metabolites (breakdown products left in the system by the medication) or has only weak metabolites. Also use medications that don't stay in your system or the baby's blood for a long time.

e. With regard to points b and d, I caution against switching a medication, that is, using one in pregnancy and another one postpartum, because this is will increase infant exposure.

3. Infant factors

a. Premature or newborn infants who have compromised kidney function and immature metabolisms are less likely than babies born at term or infants who are older to tolerate drugs in the breast milk.

b. If you supplement breast-feeding with bottle-feeding, the baby will receive less medication and there will be less exposure.

c. If infants or babies have medical conditions, the advisability of breast-feeding while taking medication should be discussed with your doctor.

NURSING STRATEGIES

1. Avoid nursing at times of peak concentration of medication. With Zoloft, for example, this would be eight to nine hours after ingestion of medicine.

2. Take your medication immediately before the infant's longest sleep period or immediately after nursing.

3. Discontinue breast-feeding if you notice that the infant is showing any signs of toxicity. Your health is important and you need to continue taking the medication, but you should not expose the baby any further.

4. Always try to get a second opinion if you're not happy or satisfied with your doctor.

5. Remember that even while you're breast-feeding, you may become pregnant if you don't use contraception. Breast-feeding is not a contraceptive method.

Adapted from the *Clinical Pharmacy Bulletin,* published by the British Columbia Children's & Women's Pharmacy, Therapeutics and Nutrition Committee.

The News Is Good—and Getting Better

The good news is that over the past four decades increasing numbers of women have been nursing their babies while taking medication. To date, there have been no reports of any major or long-lasting complications associated with any of these medications, and, as time goes by, more and more data are becoming available.

Even ten years ago, if a woman had come to me and said that she didn't want to take medication because she was going to breast-feed her baby, I would have agreed to allow her to do that. Since that time, however, my colleagues and I have learned a great deal more about the risks of exposing infants to psychotropic medications through the breast milk as well as the risks of allowing depression to go untreated. I now understand that it would be much riskier—both for the mother and for her baby—to discontinue medication postpartum.

IO

Nonpharmacological Treatments

In addition to the various medications described in Chapter 8, there is an equally wide variety of therapies not involving medications that can be used either alone or in conjunction with psychotropic drugs to manage depression and the other anxiety disorders that often accompany it. Like medications, each one will be more or less effective on particular types of depression and anxiety disorders.

Psychological Support

Although, as we have seen, depression both during pregnancy and postpartum is almost certainly related to changes in hormones and brain chemistry, it is equally important to address the psychosocial factors that have been shown to put some women more at risk than others. To do that requires not only medical but also psychological therapy. There is, in fact, some evidence that ongoing psychotherapy will actually reduce the chance of future depressive episodes, and there is certainly abundant research to indicate that it helps to prevent as well as to treat acute depression during pregnancy and in the postpartum period.

The traditional image many people have of talk therapy is of some-one lying on a couch, dredging up memories from childhood, while a bearded doctor sits in a chair behind the patient's head, almost totally silent and certainly out of sight. In fact, however, most psychotherapists dealing with an acutely depressed patient who needs help coping on a day-to-day basis not only will interact with the patient but also will ini-tially focus on the present in order to help the patient solve his or her immediate problem. Then, once the acute phase of the illness is over and the patient is more stable, they will begin to look into unresolved issues from the past that may have contributed to the current symp-toms.

In general, psychotherapy has three specific aims with relation to helping a patient through the emotional upheaval associated with de-pression:

- It aims to understand the behaviors and emotions that may con-tribute to the depressive state.
- It addresses life events such as loss, divorce, and health issues that may contribute to depression, and it helps the patient understand and gain the ability to solve or improve the situation.
- It helps the patient learn how to cope with difficult situations by providing techniques and skill sets for problem solving so that she or he will feel more empowered and in control of life.

Choosing a Therapist

Once you and your primary care doctor have agreed that treatment is necessary, you will need to discuss what kind of treatment that will be. Particularly with relation to antenatal and postpartum depression, there may be a great deal of uncertainty on your part, as well as feelings of guilt and shame related to the stigma that is still attached to psychiatric illness. For these reasons, it's important that you have a clear picture of the kinds of treatment available to you as well as of the individuals who may provide it.

Therapists come from several different backgrounds, each requiring a particular type of training, and as a result, the type of therapy each of them offers will also be different. A therapist may be a psychiatrist, that is, a medical doctor with special training in psychiatry; a psychologist, one who has a Ph.D. in the field of psychology; your general family physician; a social worker, someone with a master's degree or a doctorate in social work; or a nurse counselor who has a master's degree with training in counseling psychology. It's important to check your potential therapist's credentials because there are a lot of lay people who refer to themselves as therapists, but you want to receive help from someone with the proper training.

It would therefore be prudent to identify, with the help of your family physician or obstetrician, the kind of therapy that is best for your particular situation and to receive a recommendation for a qualified counselor. Your decision should be based on an assessment of the following issues:

- What kind of background does the therapist have? What type of therapy does she or he practice? Am I comfortable with this kind of therapy?
- How long is the treatment expected to last? How often will I see the therapist, and how long is each session?
- Is my therapist certified? Does she or he hold a valid certification in one of the particular aspects of health care listed above?
- If so, is the therapist a specialist in pregnancy-related and postpartum depression? Does she or he have a bias one way or the other about prescribing medication during these periods?
- Will my therapist consult and work with my psychiatrist, obstetrician, and/or family doctor? If the therapist is not licensed to prescribe medication, will she or he work with a doctor who is?
- What does the therapist charge, and will the cost be covered by my medical insurance—either completely or in part?
- Do I feel comfortable with this person?

The Therapeutic Relationship Is Key

It is absolutely essential that you feel comfortable with the person who is treating you; if you are not able to build a relationship based on mutual trust, chances are that you will not achieve a positive outcome.

The relationship between patient and therapist is an alliance—in fact, it is technically termed a "therapeutic alliance," which means that you are working together toward a mutual goal. It is important that you be an active participant in your own therapy and that you comply with the treatment laid out by your therapist. The treatment can take time—many weeks, if not months—and if you are not motivated, if you don't keep your appointments, you will be likely to relapse. For your therapy to be optimally effective you need to:

- Attend all your scheduled appointments
- Make the time and effort necessary to see your therapist regularly
- Maintain a positive attitude toward your sessions with your therapist

Psychotherapy, Pharmacotherapy, or Both?

Unfortunately, there is no simple, clear-cut answer to the question of whether the best choice for any given patient is psychotherapy, pharmacotherapy, or both. Chances are that if your referring physician is biased against the use of prescription medications during pregnancy, she or he will refer you to a therapist who doesn't use them. On the other hand, if the physician is a believer in medication, she or he might refer you to a psychopharmacologist, who dispenses medication. I've seen patients who were treated without medication and who did not improve, but I've also seen many women who were frustrated because they were simply handed a prescription for an antidepressant or a mood stabilizer without being offered any additional form of treatment. I would hope that the more clinicians learn about antenatal depression, the more likely they will be to set aside any prejudice they might have and prescribe the best treatment for their patients. For some women, psychotherapy alone will be enough; others will require medication in conjunction with some type of psychotherapy. What's important is that the patient is aware of all the options available to her.

The Many Faces of Psychotherapy

The forms of psychotherapy generally used to treat pregnant and lactating mothers fall into one of several categories: individual (one-on-one) and group therapy, marital/family therapy, and other forms of psychotherapies. Individual therapy may be further divided into cognitive behavior therapy (CBT), interpersonal therapy (IPT), psychodynamic therapy, and supportive psychotherapy. In groups, a mixture of techniques including CBT and IPT may be used.

COGNITIVE BEHAVIOR THERAPY (CBT)

Among the forms of individual therapy, cognitive behavior therapy is one of those most frequently used to treat pregnant and postpartum women. It combines two types of therapy—cognitive and behavioral—to help people suffering from depression and anxiety identify and change inaccurate perceptions of themselves and/or the world around them.

In cognitive therapy one learns how certain *thinking* patterns may be contributing to one's distress. It gives one insight into how one's distorted thinking can make one depressed or anxious and examines how this thinking, in turn, propels one to engage in certain types of actions that cause even more distress.

Behavioral therapy helps one to understand the connections between troublesome situations and one's reaction—which might be fear, depression, or self-damaging behavior—to those situations.

The combination (CBT) directs the patient's attention to both the right and wrong assumptions she might be making about herself and others in order to help her establish new patterns of thinking and behaving.

CBT is an active form of therapy in which the patient and her therapist work jointly to solve the patient's problems. In many ways it is like being educated, tutored, or coached by an expert. It is an extremely focused type of treatment in which the therapist gives the patient "homework" or take-home assignments and sometimes even reading materials to help speed her progress. The therapy generally requires the patient to complete twelve to sixteen weekly sessions, and some therapists may recommend two or more sessions per week if the patient is in crisis. It has proven to be extremely effective for helping to alleviate the symptoms of depression, several types of anxiety disorders, as well as eating disorders.

CBT helps the patient change her attitudes, her ways of thinking, and, above all, her behavior in the present without delving into their underlying causes. It is recommended for people who think and behave in ways that either trigger or perpetuate depression accompanied by symptoms of anxiety. It can be used either in conjunction with antidepressant medications or on its own, and it is therefore the form of therapy we recommend for patients with depression complicated by anxiety disorders.

In a study where no medications were given, Dr. Henri Chabrol and colleagues at the Université de Toulouse–Le Mirail, France, divided forty-eight new mothers with postpartum depression into three random groups. The first group received five weeks of CBT treatment, the second received eight weeks of CBT, and the third (the control group) received no treatment at all. What the researchers found was that the recovery rate was much higher for those who were treated for either five or eight weeks of CBT than it was for those who were not treated at all.

In another study, however, Dr. Peter Cooper at the University of Reading, England, compared the efficacy of four types of treatment for postpartum depression. One group of women received routine primary care, another received general counseling with no specific direction, a third received CBT, and a fourth received psychodynamic therapy. Initially, the women in the third and fourth groups fared better than the others, but after nine months the positive benefits of their treatment were no longer apparent.

Most of the research to date in the perinatal population has, in fact, concentrated on assessing the efficacy of CBT in the postpartum period.

The study that is quoted most frequently was conducted by Dr. Louis Appleby at the University of Manchester in England and compared the efficacy of pharmacological treatment with Prozac (fluoxetine) with that of CBT in a variety of combinations. One group received Prozac and one counseling session; the second received Prozac and six counseling sessions; a third group had one counseling session and no Prozac; and the final group had no Prozac and six counseling sessions. All four groups improved, but those who received Prozac fared considerably better than those who did not. And those who received six counseling sessions did better than those who received only one. What this study indicates is that both medication and counseling are effective but that counseling in conjunction with medication is more effective than counseling alone.

In my own hospital, we have studied the benefits of Paxil (paroxetine) alone as opposed to Paxil given in conjunction with twelve sessions of behavioral therapy with a Ph.D. psychologist. Personally, I was surprised to find that those who received medication without accompanying psychotherapy did just as well as those who received both.

That said, however, and despite any other research findings, both pregnant and postpartum patients in my hospital have benefited from CBT.

Kristen, for example, had already been taking four different antidepressant medications with very little relief of her symptoms when she became pregnant and started to experience severe panic attacks as well as obsessions and compulsions. She then began a course of twelve sessions with a therapist specializing in CBT and did quite well throughout the remainder of her pregnancy. In the postpartum period, however, she again became severely depressed and began to wash her hands obsessively. At that point, she agreed to take 350 mg of Effexor XR (venlafaxine) on a trial basis while continuing her CBT, which would now focus on postpartum issues. After four weeks, she began to respond to the medication and therapy, and after four months she was finally free of her crippling symptoms of anxiety.

Dory is another woman whose obsessive-compulsive symptoms increased after she gave birth to her second child and who was helped by

CBT. Although she didn't at first volunteer the information, Dory had been experiencing mild obsessive-compulsive symptoms since the age of twelve, when she checked and rechecked doorknobs, stove knobs, and shower knobs to be sure they were locked or turned off. But because her compulsions didn't really impinge upon her life, she never thought very much about them. Now, however, she had developed a more dangerous and debilitating compulsion—playing computer games.

She would close herself in her study and play for hours, totally ignoring her crying infant and restless three-year-old. Eventually her obsession increased to the point where the computer became her first love and no amount of cajoling on the part of her confused and distraught husband could coax her away from it. Dory herself was ashamed and embarrassed by her behavior but was nevertheless completely unable to control it. After twelve sessions of CBT, however, and without medication, she was able to cut down on the time she spent at her games and resume the normal tasks and behaviors of motherhood.

INTERPERSONAL PSYCHOTHERAPY (IPT)

This type of therapy assumes that the patient is ill and requires treatment, with little or no concern for assigning blame either to her or to anyone else. The treatment focuses on improving communication skills and self-esteem in order to foster the patient's sense of self and thus facilitate better behaviors and social interactions with family and friends. It is specifically useful for those whose depression is caused by mourning or grief, relationship conflicts, major life events, or social isolation. The treatment generally lasts for three to four months and concentrates on the following areas:

- Treating feelings of loss, bereavement, and grief by facilitating new relationships and helping the patient to compensate for the loss that has occurred
- Resolving or ending negative relationships involving conflict or role disputes with loved ones or significant others
- Easing the stress of transitions and changes that threaten self-esteem by empowering the patient to develop new roles and resolve conflicts

- Ending or changing unsatisfying interpersonal relationships by reducing social isolation, building new social skills, and helping the patient maintain supportive relationships

As we've seen, the lack of a supportive spouse or partner puts pregnant and postpartum women at significantly increased risk for depression; conversely, depression at these times is certain to put additional stress on the relationship. The anticipation of and adjustment to parenthood require major role transitions for both parents, and while some people appear to adjust happily and easily, others do not.

Dr. Meg Spinelli of Columbia University was one of the first to examine the effectiveness of interpersonal psychotherapy in the treatment of pregnant women. In her initial pilot study she treated thirteen women and found that IPT significantly reduced their symptoms of depression and that none of them experienced postpartum depression. These findings were so encouraging that she then went on to do a larger controlled clinical trial comparing interpersonal psychotherapy to parenting education as tools for alleviating antenatal depression. The study participants received sixteen weekly sessions lasting forty-five minutes each, and once again, those who received IPT experienced significant improvement in mood as compared to those who received parenting education. In addition, Dr. Spinelli found a significant correlation between maternal mood and mother-infant interaction. As a result, she concluded that IPT is an effective tool for treating depression, especially in pregnant women.

In another study Dr. Michael O'Hara and colleagues in the Department of Psychology at the University of Iowa provided women who were five months postpartum with twelve weekly sessions of interpersonal therapy given by a psychologist specifically trained in IPT. Once again the therapy was shown to reduce depressive symptoms and increase social adjustment.

This type of therapy, then, appears to be a good choice for women who are reluctant to expose either the baby they are carrying or the infant they are breast-feeding to antidepressant medications. For those who choose this route, however, it's important to find a therapist specifically trained in IPT who can tailor the treatment specifically to the problems of pregnant and/or postpartum women. One who did choose it and fared very well was Valerie, an accomplished pianist who recognized that she'd had problems with interpersonal relationships from a very early age.

Valerie believed that in order to survive and make her needs known she had to be aggressive and confrontational, and as she matured, her confrontational style of social interaction became more and more pronounced. Although her aggressiveness was an issue when she married, both she and her husband assumed she would mellow with time. Unfortunately, however, that didn't happen. During her pregnancy she used relaxation exercises and massage therapy to curb her anger and aggression, and her efforts were generally effective until after she gave birth. Once the baby was born, however, she became even more irritable and was, as her husband described it, "flying off the handle" at the least provocation.

She'd been referred to me by her family physician with a diagnosis of postpartum depression, and I believed that the issue of how she handled interpersonal relationships would have to be addressed immediately. I started her on 12.5 mg of Paxil CR, then increased the dose to 25 mg, at which level her symptoms of depression were under control. At that point I referred Valerie to a clinical nurse specialist at the hospital for twelve sessions of interpersonal psychotherapy. In therapy she acquired the tools she needed to communicate and handle conflict more effectively and pleasantly.

With the combination of medication and psychotherapy, her mood was stabilized and she acquired the skill sets that allowed her to modify negative behaviors she'd been practicing for many years.

PSYCHODYNAMIC PSYCHOTHERAPY

In recent years, time-consuming and expensive psychoanalysis has largely been replaced by short-term psychodynamic psychotherapy which addresses the repetitive negative patterns in a patient's life that are responsible for specific interpersonal problems. The therapy, which usually takes ten to twelve sessions, seeks to link present behaviors to core conflicts that may have occurred earlier in the patient's life.

Although it doesn't specifically focus on symptoms of depression, psychodynamic psychotherapy is useful—usually in combination with medication—for treating depression in pregnant or postpartum women for whom a family history of abandonment, neglect, or abuse may be interfering with various aspects of their ability to mother. That was exactly the scenario for Deirdre, a sweet, outwardly calm young physiotherapist who appeared to have life totally under control.

Deirdre's pregnancy was planned and proceeded uneventfully, but once her baby was born her life took a turn for the worse. At first she was able to deal with the infant's crying, but as time went on, she found herself increasingly irritated and impatient with the baby's fussing. Then, when the child became a toddler and started to assert his independence, Deirdre was diagnosed with mild to moderate depression and referred to a psychologist for psychodynamic or exploratory therapy. Psychodynamic therapy is a modern adaptation of Freud's original psychoanalytic theory, while exploratory therapy has a more interpersonal focus. Both, however, seek to understand the patient's current behaviors in light of early life experiences.

What Deirdre came to understand in therapy was that the more her baby tried to separate from her physically, the less she felt in control. Furthermore, she was able to see that these feelings were similar to those she had experienced as a child. It appears that Deirdre herself had been known as a nonconforming "naughty" child whose mother had beaten her with a wooden spoon and told her repeatedly that she was a challenge to raise. Now she kept hearing that voice in her head, until she began to confuse herself with her mother. At one point, when her baby absolutely would not listen, she found herself reaching for the wooden kitchen spoon, and that was when she realized she was repeating the very behavior she'd been struggling against all her life. That new understanding was the first step toward acquiring the skills she would need to change her negative behaviors.

GROUP THERAPY

Six or more people meet as a group with one or two leaders or facilitators to share their problems and experiences. By doing that, members of the group are able to receive validation for what they've been experiencing and to understand that their problems are not unique.

Various psychotherapeutic modes, including cognitive behavior and interpersonal therapies, are used in the group setting and have proved helpful both for alleviating postpartum depression and as an intervention for preventing it in pregnant women who are found to be at risk.

In one study, for example, Mary Morgan, an occupational therapist in Australia, provided a group of postnatally depressed women with eight group sessions and a single one-on-one session for each couple. The women-only sessions addressed a variety of problems, including anxieties surrounding the women's feelings toward their partners, their mothers, and their infants, while the couples' session focused on providing support for the father, which helped to decrease tensions between the partners. All the sessions were found to be helpful by both the women and their partners.

One form of group therapy devised by Dawn Gruen, a Seattle social worker who specialized in conducting group therapy with postpartum women, identified lack of social support, negative thoughts, and a poor marriage as potential predictors of postpartum depression and went on to develop a three-phase model of group treatment for these postpartum women. In phase one the group focuses on education and information, cognitive restructuring, and stress-reduction techniques, and the women learn strategies for developing a support system. Phase two introduces an interpersonal focus that helps to build self-esteem, and phase three concentrates on dealing with, accepting, and resolving the grief of unmet expectations surrounding the birth and parenting. Dr. Doris Ugarriza of the University of Miami collected pilot data on this promising treatment approach and found that the intervention did have an extremely positive effect on the participants' mood.

Other studies, however, indicate that instituting group therapy *during* pregnancy can actually help to *prevent* postpartum depression. One, conducted by Dr. Caron Zlotnick of Brown University, assigned thirty-seven pregnant women with at least one risk factor for postpartum depression to four sessions of group intervention using interpersonal psychotherapy. Three months after giving birth, the women who had participated in the group sessions showed no evidence of depression as compared to 33 percent of those who had been identified as at-risk but who had received no treatment. And in another study, Dr. Sandra Elliott at the University of Greenwich in England offered a sample of pregnant women group psychoeducation focusing on parenting and social support with a psychologist and a "birth visitor" (a person trained to offer support after birth in the United Kingdom). Three months after their babies were born, these women showed much less evidence of postpartum depression than those in the control group, who had not received antenatal support.

What Zlotnick's and Elliott's studies indicate is that instituting therapy—particularly interpersonal psychotherapy—during pregnancy (even when there are no overt symptoms of depression) can help women to cope successfully with the transition to motherhood and significantly reduce their chances of suffering postpartum depression.

Group therapy can be particularly helpful to women who are socially isolated and have no one with whom to share their distress. The group environment actually functions to create a "family" whom they can trust and in whom they can confide without feeling ashamed, being embarrassed, or fearing that they will be belittled. This can be especially useful for postpartum women who constantly doubt themselves and struggle to understand the skills associated with mothering.

There may, however, be barriers that make it difficult for some women to attend group therapy. Dr. Ugarriza's study, for example, noted that for some postpartum women, any kind of treatment intervention can be seen as "just one more thing" to fit into an already hectic schedule. Some women prefer to come in the evenings, when their partners can watch their children, and at my hospital we've been trying to offer child care to patients who come for treatment. We as health care providers must, I believe, do whatever we can to facilitate women's participation in this kind of therapy because of the important benefits it can provide.

Finally, in addition to actual therapy groups, there are peer groups throughout the United States and Canada that can be extremely helpful to women who are feeling isolated and alone with their problems.

My own hospital works closely with an organization called the Pacific Postpartum Society. The society offers telephone support to pregnant and postpartum women and their families, and runs information nights for partners as well as workshops, lectures, and training programs for interested groups and professionals. They also have peer support group sessions for women, run by trained facilitators.

MARITAL/COUPLES AND FAMILY THERAPY

Another form of psychotherapy that can greatly benefit pregnant and postpartum women involves the patient and her partner or the patient and one or two family members. Couples therapy seeks to change ineffective or damaging patterns of communication and to help both partners understand why their conflicts or differences occur so that they can change their behavior, increase their degree of intimacy, and in general improve the relationship.

Family therapy works to help the depressed woman's close family members understand what she is going through and how they can help. Having the understanding and support of her family can encourage the patient to stick with her treatment and practice the coping skills she is learning in psychotherapy so that her chances of a good outcome will be greatly improved.

It can be very difficult for anyone who has not experienced depression to fathom the kind of hopelessness it inflicts upon its victims. Being able to learn about the illness and identifying constructive ways of supporting their loved one can be of tremendous value to the patient's partner, her family, and the patient herself.

Alternative Interventions

All of the modes of therapy discussed so far involve multiple sessions with a trained psychotherapist, but there are alternative forms of intervention that have also proved to be effective for alleviating the stress, anxiety, and isolation that can put women at risk for antenatal or postpartum depression.

Sometimes simply becoming better educated and more familiar with the expectations and skills of parenting can make a significant difference. A study conducted by Drs. R. E. and K. K. Gordon in 1960 found that pregnant women who participated with their partners in just two educational classes focusing on child care issues during pregnancy experienced much less emotional upset six months postpartum than did those in the control group, who did not attend classes.

In my own program, we offer a parenting education group that consists of five weekly one-hour sessions. At each session we introduce one new technique, such as understanding your child, gaining cooperation, listening and talking to your child, disciplining, and dealing with sibling rivalry, and participants have the opportunity to practice their skills and share solutions with one another.

In addition to formal classes, however, sometimes having the advice and support of someone who is experienced in the birthing and mothering process will provide a woman with the confidence she needs to weather the physical and emotional ups and downs of pregnancy and new motherhood. Throughout North America that kind of support is more and more often being given by trained practitioners such as doulas and midwives.

Midwives are licensed registered nurses who have received additional training in delivering babies as well as providing antenatal and postpartum care. In the households of ancient Greece, the doula was the most important female figure, the one who helped the lady of the house through childbearing. In modern times, the term has come to mean a woman experienced in childbirth who provides continuing physical, emotional, and informational support to the mother before, during, and just after birth. Many women are now hiring trained doulas to coach them through labor, accompany them into the delivery room, and help them adjust to motherhood. Even if they have supportive spouses or significant others willing to fill this role, my patients say that having the doula makes the process less stressful and allows them to feel freer about expressing their anxiety.

How to Decide

As we have seen, there are a variety of psychological interventions and support systems available; each woman will have to decide, in consultation with her primary care physician, which one or ones would be most beneficial. Clearly, however, any woman who experiences anxiety in conjunction with pregnancy or who has been identified as at risk for postpartum depression can only benefit from finding the right kind of psychological support to see her through the transition to motherhood—even if she does not exhibit symptoms of depression.

Biological Support

Light Therapy

In Chapter 2 we discussed the fact that seasonal affective disorder (SAD) is one of the ways depression often manifests in women, and that bright-light therapy is one of the ways to relieve the condition. Although we're not quite sure how or why it works, we do know that when bright light enters the eyes it triggers the pineal gland, located in the brain, to decrease its production of the hormone melatonin. When there is no bright light, melatonin production increases, which in turn causes drowsiness. In addition, the body has its own internal clock, or circadian rhythm, that controls fluctuations in body temperature, hormone secretion, and sleep patterns. Your circadian rhythm can be either delayed or speeded up by exposure to light.

To be effective, bright-light therapy uses between 7,000 and 10,000 lux (a unit of intensity) of light, which is far greater than that produced by normal indoor artificial light. Dr. Dan Oren of Yale University published a study in 2002 in which a group of sixteen pregnant depressed women were treated with three to five weeks of bright-light therapy, and he reported that after three weeks of treatment the depression rating improved for fourteen of the participants. In a second, more controlled study published in 2004, Dr. Neill Epperson, also of Yale, selected at random ten women with major depressive disorder during pregnancy to receive either five weeks of bright-light therapy with 7,000 lux of light with an option of extending the treatment to ten weeks, or placebo (treatment with only 500 lux). At ten weeks the effects of the bright-light treatment were better than at five weeks, with complete remission of depressive symptoms. The researchers concluded once again that light therapy appeared to be an effective way of treating antenatal depression.

Dr. Maria Corral, a reproductive psychiatrist in our program and one of the pioneers in this type of treatment, has systematically conducted studies that show the efficacy of bright-light therapy for alleviating the symptoms of seasonal postpartum depression.

Bright-light therapy is an appealing and—based on the research— apparently viable form of therapy for pregnant women and postpartum breast-feeding women who are reluctant to expose their babies to medications. It's easy to use, available at home, and doesn't require women to travel to therapy sessions. It should, however, be undertaken with the guidance of a medical specialist who knows how to use the treatment properly.

The Importance of Self-Care

Whatever form of therapy a woman chooses to help alleviate her depression, particularly postpartum, self-care is always a critical component of ensuring her well-being. In their book *Women's Moods*, Dr. Deborah Sichel and Jeanne Driscoll refer to the aspects of this self-nurturing by using the acronym NURSE—nutrition and needs, understanding, rest and relaxation, spirituality, and exercise.

It's very easy for any new mother to be so concerned about meeting her baby's needs that she fails to take care of her own. Finding the time to take care of herself may, however, be one of the simplest as well as one of the most important things she can do to avoid or alleviate the symptoms of postpartum depression. These days many women are looking to complementary or alternative medicine for their preferred modes of treatment and self-nurturing. Although alternative medicine is not my particular area of expertise, I would like to share what I know about the efficacy as well as the potential contraindications of some of the most popular treatments, with the caveat that any woman seeking one of these treatments first consult with a reliable practitioner to be sure that it is appropriate for her.

HERBAL TREATMENTS

Herbal medicine is an ancient tradition in both India and China, and it is currently amassing an increasing number of followers in the Western world as well.

There are a number of herbs known to have an effect on mood, anxiety, and insomnia, but one of the most popular and also the most widely researched is St. John's wort. In a study published in the *British Medical Journal* in 1996, a group of researchers analyzed twenty-three randomized trials involving fifteen hundred patients and found it to be significantly more effective than either no medication or placebo for treating mild to moderate depression. A second, French study also found it to be useful. At least two other studies, however, have found it not to be an effective treatment for moderate to major depression.

Currently, one of the problems associated with its use by postpartum mothers is that there have been no studies to indicate how much, if any, of the herb is passed into the breast milk. In addition, it induces the manufacture in the body of monoamine oxidase, an enzyme that can interact with antidepressant medication and potentially cause serotonin toxicity, the symptoms of which include agitation, excitement, tremors, altered mental state, and fever. For both these reasons, I don't recommend it as a primary or adjunct treatment of either pregnancy-related or postpartum depression.

In addition to St. John's wort, there are many remedies used in the practice of Chinese herbal medicine for the treatment of depression. Although modern, contaminant-free versions of the traditional herbs are now being manufactured in the United States and several other Western countries, there are still no studies to show that they are effective for the treatment of depression and no data with regard to their safety for either mother or child. So, again, I would be concerned for any woman who chose the herbal path while pregnant or breast-feeding.

Omega-3 Fatty Acids

Although much has been written about the benefits of getting sufficient amounts of omega-3s in our diet, either by increasing our consumption of fish (particularly salmon) or by taking a dietary supplement, the jury is still out on whether or not they have a beneficial effect in the treatment of major depression. Although there is some evidence to indicate a positive effect, the one study done with relation to pregnant women found them not to be efficacious at all.

Massage Therapy

This is one age-old practice whose efficacy I have seen for myself and that I think has been much undervalued in Western countries. It is a part of the traditional "lying-in time" in many cultures, including my native India. Each year when I go back home, I visit with postpartum women at home as well as in nursing homes and hospitals and am constantly reminded of how much beneficial time off they receive at this critical juncture in their lives. Traditionally in India both mothers and infants are massaged regularly, and in fact, I massaged my own babies until they were six months of age. I believe that it would be impossible to overestimate the value of the closeness achieved through this kind of touch and that children who have been touched in this way at a very young age will continue to use touch as a way of demonstrating affection.

Although there have been no clinical trials demonstrating the efficacy of touch as a mode of healing, Dr. Tiffany Field of the Touch Research Institute at the University of Miami, Florida, did a study comparing the benefits of massage with the benefits of relaxation therapy in thirty-two depressed teenage mothers and found that those who received massage therapy showed significantly positive changes in behavior as well as reduced levels of cortisol found in the saliva, while those who received relaxation therapy showed no change at all.

In addition, in a separate study, Dr. Field found that massaging their babies was more efficacious than rocking for relieving stress and anxiety in the mothers. And the babies who were massaged not only cried less but slept more and were generally calmer than those who were not massaged.

ACUPUNCTURE

Acupuncture is yet another traditional Chinese medical practice that has found popularity in the West. Research has shown that it is an effective treatment for many psychological problems including depression, there are no contraindications, and it does not interfere with conventional antidepressant therapy or with lactation. In one particular study conducted by Dr. D. Tao and colleagues where traditional Chinese medicine practitioners evaluated patients, it was shown to be beneficial for alleviating chronic anxiety and depression. To date, however, there have been no studies evaluating the usefulness of acupuncture specifically in treating depressed pregnant and/or postpartum women.

Inpatient Therapy

In England more than fifty years ago, Dr. T. Main introduced the idea of hospitalizing the infant along with the mother if the mother required hospitalization for a psychiatric illness, in order to avoid the negative consequences of separation. I include this kind of inpatient service among alternative forms of treatment because it is still not widely available to most women. Since Dr. Main first put forward the idea, mother-baby units have been established in only a few countries, including the United Kingdom, Australia, and New Zealand, and more recently at my hospital, BC Women's in Canada. At the moment we have only one bed in the obstetrical unit available to pregnant or postpartum women with psychiatric illnesses and their babies. Presently, we are the only hospital in the country to offer this service at all, so we are very proud of the progress we've made.

Fourteen years ago, when my patient Morgan was hospitalized with symptoms of bipolar illness after the birth of her son, Bill, babies were not allowed to stay with their mothers in these situations because it was feared that they would not be safe. We had to sneak the baby into her room (something we still discuss when she comes every six months to have her lithium levels and kidney function checked), and to this day she is grateful for the opportunity I was able to give her, even when she was quite ill, to bond with her infant. Thankfully, sneaking around is no longer necessary at my hospital, but throughout the rest of Canada and the United States it still remains an issue.

The rationale for mother-baby units is quite simple. Experts agree that no mother should be separated from her infant for any prolonged period of time. In fact, when a baby requires hospitalization, the mother is generally allowed to sleep in the child's room and continue to remain an active caregiver along with the nurses and doctors. It stands to reason, then, that the reverse should also be true, if supervised properly.

Studies have shown that even a brief separation from the mother during the first year of life can have negative consequences for the infant, including listlessness, avoidance, excessive crying, and difficulties achieving intimacy. For the mother, hospitalization in a psychiatric unit can be embarrassing and stigmatizing and, as a result, can actually become a barrier to her recovery.

Although I don't mean to be an alarmist or to indicate that separation from one's infant for a few days or even a few weeks is going to cause permanent damage to either mother or child, I do want to let people know that an alternative to such separation does exist in many countries and that this is an area where we in North America may not be as enlightened as we would like to consider ourselves.

Consider the Big Picture

As you can see, there are many kinds of nonpharmacological intervention and support available to women who are depressed either during pregnancy or postpartum. While I believe that the benefits of antidepressant medications far outweigh their risks, I do understand that some women will still prefer not to expose either themselves or their babies to these drugs. If that is the case, I cannot stress strongly enough that it is important to seek some kind of psychotherapy, either alone or in conjunction with other forms of support, to see you through and help manage and/or alleviate your symptoms. The most detrimental and dangerous thing any woman can do, for herself, her baby, and her family, is to allow her depression to go untreated. For more information on the various kinds of support that may be available to you, please see Resources, page 251.

11

When Depression Goes Untreated, It Affects the Unborn Child

In the opening paragraph of *David Copperfield* Charles Dickens writes, "To begin my life with the beginning of my life, I record that I was born," indicating that the author believed life began at birth. Since Dickens's time, there has been much philosophical debate about whether life begins at conception, when the fetal heart begins to beat, when the fetus is considered viable, or when the baby is born.

It's certainly not the business of this book to enter into that never-ending debate, but as a physician who works with pregnant women every day, I know that my patients feel they are carrying a life inside them. They wonder what their baby will look like—does it have blue eyes like its father, red hair like its mother, its grandmother's nose? Is it swimming around in a pool of amniotic fluid having a great old time? And they instinctively want to protect that life at all costs; it is precious, and they would do anything in their power to keep it from harm.

This is a powerful attachment that begins almost at the moment of conception and continues throughout the life of the child, no matter how long that life might be. And because it is so powerful, the way the mother imagines and fantasizes about the child she is carrying has a profound impact upon the psychological and physiological development of the fetus itself.

Somehow we have always known this, and even in ancient times, when there was no sophisticated imaging technique to allow us to visualize the fetus, it was understood that the mother's negative emotions had an adverse effect on her unborn child. For example, it was believed in one culture that being startled by a leaping hare would cause the mother to give birth to a baby with a harelip. In another the belief was that if the mother washed clothes in a river full of fish, her child might develop a scaly skin condition known as ichthyosis.

Depression and Its Effect on Fetal Attachment

Kelly Lindgren of the Madison School of Nursing in Madison, Wisconsin, studied 252 adult pregnant women between twenty and forty weeks of gestation to determine the association among maternal-fetal attachment, prenatal depression, and health practices during pregnancy. Her findings showed that women who were not depressed were more likely to engage in healthy behaviors (such as not smoking, not drinking, not using illicit drugs, and obtaining proper prenatal care) and that these behaviors were predictive of a better maternal-fetal attachment than the less healthy behaviors of those who were depressed.

Professor M. S. Cranley at the University of Buffalo School of Nursing has described the maternal-fetal attachment as "the extent to which the woman engages in behaviors that represent an affiliation and interaction with her unborn child." In other words, the way an expectant mother acts and feels is indicative of the degree to which she is bonding with the fetus. The stronger she feels herself, the more attached she will be to her baby. If she is relaxed and enjoying her pregnancy, the fetus will also be relaxed and will grow into a happy infant and, ultimately, a well-adjusted human being.

To demonstrate that link scientifically, Dr. Leo Leader at the University of New South Wales in Sydney, Australia, showed one group of pregnant women the emotionally charged film *Sophie's Choice*, while a control group viewed a neutral film that would not cause emotional upset. Leader and his colleagues were able to demonstrate through the use of a fetal heart monitor that the fetal heartbeat increased as the women watching *Sophie's Choice* became more emotionally stressed.

Maternal Stress and the Unborn Child

It is, of course, true that no matter how hard we try to reduce our level of stress, we all still have to deal with the normal irritations of daily life—looking for a parking space, standing in line in the supermarket, beeping our way through an endless menu of options on the telephone. And the more of that kind of stress a woman encounters while she's pregnant, the greater is the chance that it will have some effect on her baby. But it's also the way she *reacts* to these stresses that helps determine the degree to which they will impact the fetus.

B. R. Van den Bergh, of the Population and Family Study Centre in Brussels, Belgium, followed seventy mother-infant pairs from the first trimester of pregnancy through the child's ninth year. Starting at thirty-six weeks of pregnancy, ultrasound imaging showed that the children of highly anxious women were hyperactive, and when they were studied at seven months after birth, these same babies tended to be "difficult," to be irritable, and to cry excessively. Nine years later, boys in particular continued to be hyperactive, to show signs of attention deficit, and to engage in aggressive behavior.

Another study, this one conducted by Dr. Lynn Groome of the University of South Alabama, also supports the evidence that the mother's psychological state affects her unborn child. Groome's study used ultrasound technology and found that the fetuses of anxious mothers spent more time in quiet sleep and exhibited less obvious body movement, particularly of the hands and feet, in active sleep than those of healthy mothers. Research on how maternal stress affects the fetus has shown both overactivity and underactivity in utero. What these findings clearly indicate is that the maternal environment does have direct effects on the developing baby—the long-term implications of both the illness and treatment methods remain to be elucidated in larger studies than are currently available. And Dr. Barry Zuckerman at Boston City Hospital, who also examined the relationship between maternal depression and infant behavior at three days after birth, found that babies born to depressed mothers cried excessively and were extremely difficult to soothe, leading him to conclude that physiological stress during pregnancy was related to adverse outcomes for the baby.

Sometimes tragic times provide science with unique opportunities. After a series of earthquakes devastated southern Italy in November 1980, researchers who used ultrasound techniques to examine the effects on twenty-eight pregnant women between eighteen and thirty-six weeks of gestation found that their fetuses had increased heart rates and periods of extreme hyperactivity lasting anywhere from two to eight hours at a time. Another study of babies born to Israeli women during the Six-Day War, which looked at their behavior shortly after birth and again two years later, found that they were—and continued to be—anxious, tense, irritable, and socially maladjusted.

Stress, Hormones, Neurotransmitters, and the Fetus

In Chapter 3 we discussed the relationship between mood, hormones, and a variety of neurotransmitters released by the brain. Among those hormones, cortisol is most closely related to stress, and it has been shown to affect not only the expectant mother but also her unborn child. Laboratory experiments have shown that creating prenatal stress in animals leads to delayed development of motor skills, impaired cognitive learning, attention deficit, maladaptive social and sexual behaviors, and increased anxiety, among other psychological and physical problems. Creating stress in monkeys by exposing them to unexpected noise in late pregnancy has also been shown to create elevated levels of cortisol in their offspring. The results of these and other studies have led some researchers to believe that human physiology may act in a similar way.

Cortisol and Fetal Stress

When the body is stressed, a cascade of reactions leading to increased levels of particular hormones occurs in the brain.

We know, for example, that when a woman's body is unusually stressed during pregnancy, the placenta produces large quantities of a hormone called CRH (corticotropin-releasing hormone), which has been shown to be associated with spontaneous preterm labor. Viviette Glover and her colleagues at the Fetal Neonatal Stress Research Group have found that levels of cortisol in the blood of pregnant women rose in response to the increased release of CRH and that fetal levels of cortisol were also increased. In other words, when stress leads to increased cortisol levels in the blood of pregnant women, that cortisol is also transferred to the fetus through the placenta.

We don't know exactly why increased CRH is associated with preterm labor, but we do know that premature birth, in and of itself, leads to a variety of problems for the newborn. In fact, the World Health Organization has identified low birth weight, intrauterine growth retardation, and premature birth as the leading causes of impaired development in newborns and infant death. A large study conducted in Brazil by Dr. Patricia de Carvalho Rondó and colleagues and replicated by Dr. Pathik Wadhwa and colleagues at the University of California found that maternal psychological factors were associated with intrauterine growth retardation, low birth weight, and prematurity.

Although low birth weight is not always related to premature birth, premature birth is almost invariably associated with low birth weight, and these two problems create a serious public health issue in the United States, where the rate of infant death is one of the highest of any developed nation, particularly among African Americans.

Neurotransmitters and Fetal Stress

In addition to increased levels of CRH, increased levels of norepinephrine in depressed pregnant women, particularly during the third trimester, may also be associated with impaired fetal development and preterm delivery. In fact, mothers with depressive symptoms in late pregnancy are 3.90 percent more likely than healthy women to deliver low-birth-weight babies, 3.02 percent more likely to have babies with impaired intra-uterine growth, and 3.39 percent more likely to deliver prematurely.

One reason for this may be that the elevated levels of norepineph-rine released in response to the mother's stress are transferred through the placenta and cause a reduction in uterine blood flow, thereby re-stricting the delivery of oxygen and nutrients to the fetus. Dr. Tiffany Field and her colleagues at the University of Miami, in Florida, tested the babies born to women with depressive symptoms and found that at birth they had increased levels of both cortisol and norepinephrine and decreased levels of dopamine and serotonin, just like their mothers. The babies also had poor motor ability, were less active and more lethargic than average, and demonstrated behaviors, such as withdrawal, that are associated with stress. Finally, when tested with electroencephalograms, they showed impairment of brain activity.

Another study, conducted by Dr. Brenda Lundy, a psychologist at the University of Miami Medical Center, also showed that babies born to depressed mothers were less physiologically developed, showed fewer interests, and demonstrated restricted facial expression compared to those born to healthy mothers. Finally, an important study completed by Dr. Jerónima Teixeira at Queen Charlotte's and Chelsea Hospital in London demonstrated that maternal anxiety in pregnancy was associ-ated with uterine artery resistance, leading to reduced blood flow to the uterus and, therefore, smaller babies, with all the complications associ-ated with low birth weight. In short, when a woman is depressed during pregnancy, the physiological changes created by her condition appear to be transferred to the fetus, leading to adverse physiological and psycho-logical outcomes for the baby.

In my own practice, I have seen how devastating these problems can be. I met Derek for the first time when he was a year old. His mother, Rena, is a stoic woman of Yugoslavian descent who had been extremely resistant to taking medications during pregnancy but had appeared to do well with intensive counseling. I later discovered, however, that she had not been truthful when reporting her symptoms because she was afraid that her doctor would, as she put it, "force medication down her throat."

When Derek turned one, Rena had a party for him and invited a group of his friends. The one-year marker was important for Rena because she was planning a second pregnancy, which is what precipitated her making an appointment to see me.

She arrived with little Derek in tow, and as we proceeded to talk about her next pregnancy, discussing the fact that she intended to stop working for four months and had "everything taken care of," I noticed that she had completely turned her back on her child, who was not yet able to walk. He was just about managing to balance himself while standing and was tugging at her skirt, crying, and effectively doing everything in his power to gain his mother's attention. Yet not for a second did Rena even turn in his direction, much less make any attempt to soothe him. Finally, I implored her to attend to Derek's needs, at which point she turned to me and said, "Dr. Misri, this happens every day, and no matter how much I try to soothe him, he just doesn't stop."

To me, that wasn't really a satisfactory response or explanation, and I recommended that she have Derek evaluated by our occupational therapist, who tested him using the Bayley Scales of Infant Development. Test results showed that he was extremely delayed in many areas, including slow motor activity, poor muscle tone, difficult temperament, and increased irritability. In the end, both the developmental pediatrician and the infant psychiatrist who were brought in to work with him strongly suggested that his poor level of functioning was related to his mother's compromised mental state both during pregnancy and following his birth. Rena did reluctantly decide to take medications during her second pregnancy, and this time, thankfully, she gave birth without complications to a healthy baby.

Untreated Depression Leads to Poor Outcomes

The results of all these studies, as well as my own clinical experience, lead to the conclusion that leaving depression untreated during pregnancy is likely to have effects on the fetus that translate to problems for the child down the road.

A study I recently conducted with my own colleagues and published in the *Canadian Journal of Psychiatry* showed that severe depression and anxiety disorders suffered by pregnant women were important contributors to the adverse outcomes of their babies. Although all women were being treated with medication, some of them relapsed in the third trimester and remained symptomatic. Afraid that their babies might be adversely affected, they declined to increase their doses and subsequently gave birth to babies who required admission to the intensive care nursery for twenty-four to forty-eight hours. The good news is that at the time of discharge, the babies were completely healthy. This study confirmed our concern that undertreated depression and anxiety in pregnancy can lead to poor baby outcomes. A large study conducted by Dr. Tony Chung at the Chinese University of Hong Kong and published in 2001 has reported similar findings. Chung and his colleagues followed 959 women from early pregnancy through birth and found that depression in late pregnancy was associated with increased admissions to a neonatal care unit.

Many researchers have concluded that these neonatal problems may be more than short-term. For example, a study conducted by Dr. David Barker in Southampton, England, followed low-birth-weight babies to adulthood and found that they suffered a higher-than-average incidence of hypertension and ischemic heart disease. Although it is not yet clear to what degree the expectant mother's psychological distress may create permanent problems for her child, what is clear is that we need to do whatever we can to reduce the degree to which pregnant women are exposed to stress and negative events, and to treat symptoms of anxiety and depression when they do occur.

12

And What About Fathers?

It may surprise you to know that in certain cultures up to 65 percent of expectant fathers experience symptoms of pregnancy when their partners are expecting. They may have food cravings, gain weight, suffer morning sickness or cramps, and even go through an occasional mood swing. In fact, these "sympathetic symptoms" are so prevalent and so well recognized that they actually have a name—Couvade syndrome, from the French *couver*, which means "to incubate."

Some men, it appears, even experience hormonal shifts similar to those of pregnant women. Two Canadian researchers, Dr. Katherine Wynne-Edwards, of Queen's University, and Dr. Anne Storey, a professor of psychology at Memorial University in Newfoundland, examined hormone levels in the blood and saliva of expectant fathers at ten weeks of their partner's pregnancy, a few weeks prior to birth, and immediately after delivery. Amazingly, they found high levels of prolactin and an increased concentration of cortisol in the men before birth and low levels of testosterone immediately after birth.

In some primitive societies men would actually go into a nearby hut and huff and puff while their wives were in labor, indicating by their grunting and groaning that they were supporting and sympathizing with the woman who was going through the birthing process. In ancient cultures—when women generally found support among the other women in their village or tribe and fathers were more or less left on the sidelines—this may, in fact, have been the only way men had of participating in pregnancy and childbirth.

In today's culture, however, things are different. Expectant dads indicate their support by attending prenatal classes, going to doctor's appointments with their partners, and by being present as coaches in the delivery room. This increased participation is certainly a good thing, but it also brings additional stress. Fathers today bear a huge burden of responsibility, and doing these things may help them to satisfy their need to identify with their pregnant partner or to overcome the feelings of jealousy that can occur because the experience of pregnancy belongs so exclusively to the woman. It is also a way to help them cope with any fears they might have about bringing a child into the world—because, whether they are willing to admit it or not, men too become anxious about their partner's pregnancy and their own impending parenthood.

Dads Need to Feel Needed

It is generally accepted that once a new baby comes into the world, the infant bonds with the new mother, and the new father may feel excluded from their solid unit of two. In reality, however, as we discussed in the previous chapter, the bond between mother and baby begins during pregnancy, and I believe that many men may experience Couvade syndrome as an expression of their desire to be part of the mother-child dyad even before the baby is born.

Recently, I saw a case of Couvade for myself when Lorraine, whom I had treated for depression during two previous pregnancies, confided her concern about her husband, Mark. During her previous pregnancies, I'd gotten to know Mark well. He was a tall, slim man who worked out regularly and was very helpful to Lorraine. In fact, he'd even come as a guest to one of our group sessions and shared his story with others in the group.

Now, in the third month of her third pregnancy, Lorraine told me that although Mark was still sympathetic toward her, he was at least forty pounds overweight, was not feeling well, had been experiencing mood swings similar to her own, and had virtually stopped participating in activities with their two- and four-year-old children.

When I saw Mark in a separate session, I realized that possibly his symptoms were an expression of Couvade syndrome. Mark was extremely honest and told me that he was feeling excluded from this third pregnancy, that he was jealous of Lorraine, and that he was very worried about having a third child because the family's finances were already stretched to the limit and they had taken a second mortgage on their house. His anxiety had been awakening him in the middle of the night, he was always tired, and he'd been unable to be sexually intimate with his wife. As a result of all this, he felt isolated, rejected, and lonely.

After hearing his story, I referred Mark to a colleague for therapy. Eventually he was able to talk through and resolve many of his anxieties and frustrations.

Mark's emotional stress was not unlike that of many men who feel left out, unappreciated, or even under siege, particularly in the postpartum period. It's not unusual for a new father to find himself thrust into a situation for which he's had no training and having to deal with a partner who appears suddenly to have turned into an angry alien. Very often, I've found, arguments occur around issues of cleanliness. Women become overly concerned with washing an older child's toys or sanitizing the entire kitchen after every meal, and no matter how much their partners try to help, they are never clean or tidy enough.

When a baby is born, roles and expectations change, and these inevitable changes can lead to unspoken tensions between partners, as they did for Rose and her husband, Gary. "I cannot believe that all she talks about is how badly I'm folding the laundry," Gary exclaimed at our first meeting. Men such as Gary often feel that their partners are too preoccupied with things that seem unimportant, while women complain that if they weren't hypercritical, the men wouldn't do anything at all. "Every time there's a mess," Rose said about Gary, "be it unwashed laundry or dirty dishes, I wonder why he can't see these things for himself. Is he blind? Can't he see there's a mess? Why do I have to harass him into doing every little thing? I even have to badger him into changing a light-bulb. Surely he can see that it's dark!" This kind of ongoing conflict can quickly become a vicious cycle, with the woman simultaneously "re-minding" the man of what needs to be done and rejecting all sugges-tions of practical help from her partner, who in turn becomes even more frustrated and hostile.

Sometimes the baby itself can become the focus of discord between partners, particularly if there's an older relative, such as a grandparent, who is constantly offering unsolicited advice and thereby driving a wedge between the parents. Even without such meddling, however, in-dividual beliefs or parenting styles can create contention between part-ners. Some people, for example, believe that it's okay to let the baby cry for a few minutes if she or he awakens at night, while others can't stand it and want to run into the nursery immediately. When parents disagree on issues such as this, it's easy for them to make the baby the innocent scapegoat for their own differences.

When the Need Becomes Too Great

If the woman is suffering from postpartum depression, the situation, from the father's point of view, can seem beyond his ability to cope. In these circumstances men bear an enormous burden, they feel that their own needs are being neglected, and no matter what they do for their partner, it isn't ever enough. As a result, many men feel emotionally drained, and all they really want is concrete, step-by-step instructions for how to "fix" the problem.

Jeff, a twenty-nine-year-old engineer, expressed these feelings most forcefully when he attended a session at my clinic to which we'd invited postpartum dads. "I just don't know what to do anymore," he said. "I come home from a stressful day at work and my wife is so irritable and upset that even a simple question like 'How was your day?' causes her to snap and burst into tears. Then she just starts screaming and saying things like 'What do you mean, what was my day like? Obviously it wasn't as productive as yours!' Am I supposed to *not* ask her about her day? I feel like I'm in a no-win situation, and I really need some help."

Help is something Roger was willing to give—and give, and give—when his wife, Brenda, underwent an acute postpartum depression following the birth of their second child. In the end, he gave so much that he, too, became depressed.

Roger and Brenda are both perfectionists, and they had established a routine for the baby's nighttime feedings that was driving them both a bit nuts. For some reason, they'd decided that the infant was a "high-maintenance baby," although she was awakening approximately every four hours, which is absolutely normal for a newborn. The problem was that Roger and Brenda wanted her to wake up *exactly* every four hours on the dot, and if she awakened five minutes early, neither of them could deal with this slight deviation from their predetermined schedule. As time went on, Brenda became more and more anxious. Her milk supply began to dry up, and eventually she gave up nursing. At that point Roger took over all the feedings, and as a result, he became so stressed and sleep-deprived that he developed a depression of his own. We are now treating him with a combination of antidepressants, antianxiety medication, and psychotherapy. I'm pleased to say he is doing quite well.

While coping with postpartum depression is always taxing for the man in the partnership, if either or both of the partners are unaware of what's really happening, the relationship is in danger of being damaged beyond repair. As a tragic example, Jackie and Wayne were both students in their twenties and married for just over two years when Jackie unexpectedly became pregnant. Neither of the young parents had any real understanding of the impact the baby would have on their lives, and shortly after Jackie gave birth, they began blaming each other for each little thing that, in their educated opinion, was going wrong: the baby was too fussy, the baby didn't sleep enough; in short, the baby just wasn't "perfect" enough. There were many reasons for their escalating arguments, but the true underlying cause was that Jackie was suffering a severe postpartum depression.

After their bickering and fighting had gone on for some time, Wayne returned from classes one day and Jackie just "went off." She began to attack him physically, screaming that *she* couldn't go to class because she had to stay home with the baby he'd "dumped" on her, and when he tried to restrain her from hitting him, she called the police. Within minutes he was in handcuffs and being led off to jail. A judge issued a restraining order on the grounds that he had physically abused his wife (which wasn't the truth), and even though Jackie later retracted the charges and apologized to her husband, the damage to their relationship had already been done and would be extremely difficult to mend.

Jackie and Wayne were both unaware of Jackie's depression until it precipitated a violent episode, but sometimes it's the father who is the first to realize that something is terribly wrong, who has to be the one to call the doctor or take his partner to the hospital, and who bears the sole responsibility for the safety of both his partner and his child. When the mother is hospitalized, it's often on an emergency basis; the stress on the father in these situations is sometimes simply too much. He may feel guilty or angry, he may try to distance himself from the situation, and more often than not he needs a tremendous amount of education and support.

For Diane, a patient of mine who was having thoughts about harming her baby, there came a point when those thoughts became so severe and continuous that her husband, Stan, phoned my office at six o'clock one morning and left a message saying that his wife was in urgent need of being seen. When the couple arrived, I saw immediately that Diane was, in fact, in danger of harming both her children, one eighteen months and the other just two months old.

She was hospitalized immediately and has now recovered completely, but if Stan hadn't made that call, I might not have known how serious her condition had become. If for no other reason than that they are so often the first ones to be aware that their partners are deteriorating, it's most important that we include fathers in any treatment plan for women who are at risk for or experiencing postpartum depression.

When Fathers Really Do Know Best

In my own practice, I always talk to the husband or partner about how to recognize depression and how to deal with a crisis should it arise. I make him aware that there is a possibility his partner might develop paranoid ideations and might even become suicidal. I emphasize the fact that he not only *can* but *should* call me in any situation he deems to be an emergency. Often, in fact, I have found that the father's input is invaluable to my treatment of postpartum mothers.

In a paper I published in the *Canadian Journal of Psychiatry* examining the importance of partner support for the treatment of postpartum depression, I concluded that simply by increasing men's awareness and creating a forum for women to discuss their feelings openly with their partners, we were helping them to recover more quickly than those who did not have an opportunity to share their experience. But the men are also in need of support, and I always recommend that postpartum dads take some time off to nurture themselves, because if they don't, they too are in danger of collapsing under the stress.

The Father as Primary Caregiver: It Can Be a Heavy Burden

Often a woman who suffers postpartum depression is barely able to function, so the new father becomes the sole support and protector of his partner and his baby (as well as older children, if there are any). Once she recovers, it is also his job to rebuild the family unit. Mary M. Meighan, a professor of nursing in Jefferson City, Tennessee, has identified the following themes in the experience of postpartum dads:

1. *"She became an alien."* They felt that their wives had changed so much they were no longer themselves.
2. *Loss of intimacy.* Husbands reported that their relationships had become "guarded and nonreciprocal."
3. *He attempted to fix the problem.* Husbands, in an attempt to help

their wives recover, sought to find the cause of the depression so that they could "fix" the problem.

4. *The relationship was altered.*

5. *He made sacrifices.* The husbands assumed increased responsibilities to care for their wife and child as well as the household and made sacrifices for the well-being of the family.

6. *There was a real crisis.* The men felt that others in their network lacked an understanding of postpartum depression and that many health care professionals minimized the problem.

7. *His world collapsed.* The sacrifices and responsibility took an emotional toll, and the husbands felt as if their world were collapsing around them.

8. *Loss of control.* The men described their world as being unpredictable and out of control.

Meighan and her colleagues also concluded that these men were inclined to suffer in silence because of the stigma attached to postpartum depression. We need to break that silence!

Advice to Postpartum Dads

This is the advice and reassurance I always give in my practice to the partners of women suffering postpartum depression:

1. *Your partner's illness is treatable. Don't be afraid of it.* Although there is still some stigma attached to it, more people now know about postpartum depression than ever before, and if you talk about it with your doctor or another health care provider, he or she will know what you're talking about. Also, you might want to go to the Web site www.postpartumdads.org, which is run by men whose partners suffered from postpartum depression, or www.postpartum. net, run by Postpartum Support International. Both are valuable resources that offer education and support to help alleviate whatever anxieties you have about the condition.

2. *Make sure you get a referral to an expert in the area where you live.* He or she may be a psychiatrist, a psychologist, a family physician, or an obstetrician trained in the area of postpartum depression, but whoever it is, you need to trust and feel comfortable with him or her.

3. *Don't be impatient with the treatment process.* It may take weeks if not months for your partner to recover. She may be irritable or depressed; she may have crying spells and be unpredictable. This is to be expected, but every week you will see positive changes and she will continue to feel better in the hands of an expert. You may need to go with your partner to talk to the doctor, because sometimes she may find it difficult to communicate openly and properly—not because she doesn't want to, but because her depression can negatively impact her ability to do so.

4. *Don't let your partner unilaterally discontinue treatment.* Once the acute phase of her depression is over, your partner may be tempted to stop her medication or treatment. Don't let this happen. In fact, she may have to continue treatment for many months after the acute episode is over in order to avoid a relapse.

5. *Don't try to "talk her out of" the depression.* Remember, depression is a disease. You wouldn't try to talk her out of a heart attack or diabetes, and depression is no different. You need to be supportive, understanding, and sympathetic—not to minimize or invalidate her illness.

6. *You have to keep your own emotions in check, difficult as it may be.* It's easy to become angry, irritated, or impatient with your partner. But this is a time when she needs your tenderness; during this time your love and support are her lifelines. Although she may not be able to ask you directly, you need to be there for her.

7. *Avoid statements such as "You look a bit down today; have you taken your Prozac?"* These kinds of comments will only make her feel worse. Remember that people who don't understand depression may look upon those who are depressed as "crazy." Your partner

already feels that way, so don't make her feel even more helpless and worthless.

8. *Do not be shy about asking for support from other members of your family.* That's what they're there for, in good times and bad. If your mother or mother-in-law is available, don't hesitate to ask for her help; you'll be surprised to see how willing she is to lend a hand.

9. *If your partner is feeling acutely suicidal or homicidal, or you feel that your baby or other children are in danger because of her illness, take her to the nearest emergency room and have her admitted.* You must do this, even though it will certainly add to your level of stress. Again, mobilize members of the family to help you out in this crisis.

10. *The good news is that your partner will recover.* She is going to come back and be a mother and a partner to you, so hang in there.

Postpartum Depression in Dads? Really?

The more I see and learn about depression both during pregnancy and in the postpartum period, the more I am becoming sensitized to the needs of postpartum dads. I now realize that fathers, too, can suffer postpartum depression. Particularly if a man has a family history of depression, this is a time of vulnerability for him, just as it is for a woman—and as it was for Fred.

Fred and his wife, Krissie, live on Vancouver Island, one of the most beautiful places in the world. When Krissie became pregnant, both she and Fred were ecstatic, and even though she suffered a period of postpartum depression, they had a great deal of help from their families and things were going well. I knew Fred because he often accompanied Krissie to her appointments with me, and after a time I began to notice that whenever we started to discuss the difficulties they were having at home, Fred became a bit teary-eyed and was clearly in some sort of emotional crisis himself.

At the end of one particular appointment, Krissie asked me to see Fred on his own because, she said, she thought he had postpartum depression. I was startled by her use of that term and impressed that even in the midst of her own problems she was aware enough to see that Fred, too, was having a rough time.

When I talked with him on his own, Fred told me that he had a family history of depression going back three generations. He also said that he'd been worried about the family's finances because Krissie hadn't been working and he'd been too dysfunctional to work efficiently himself. He also confided that recently he'd begun to have obsessive thoughts about wanting to harm his baby.

In fact, Fred was in the midst of a major depression with symptoms of obsessive-compulsive disorder, but until Krissie noticed the change in his behavior, it hadn't even occurred to him that he might be depressed.

Interestingly, Dr. Jonathan Abramowitz at the Mayo Clinic has recently published a paper documenting the acute and rapid onset of obsessive-compulsive disorder in four men coinciding with the birth of their babies. The thoughts (and in one case compulsions) he documented were strikingly similar to those normally experienced by postpartum women. In an attempt to explain this phenomenon, in a follow-up study Dr. Abramowitz and his colleagues sent a questionnaire to three hundred childbearing women and their partners, 65 percent of whom reported normal intrusive thoughts about harm somehow coming to their babies. What is most fascinating, however, is that childbirth can trigger either the onset or the worsening of OCD in men, just as it does in women. To me this means that when a man perceives childbirth as a stressful event, it can put him at risk for the disease.

Hospitalization: The Worst-Case Scenario

It should not be surprising that the greatest stress for a new father is the depression, either during or following pregnancy, of his partner. In fact, several researchers have found that a mother's postpartum depression significantly affects the mood of the father, and some studies have shown that this is also true for depression during pregnancy.

The worst-case scenario for both parents is, of course, when the mother needs to be hospitalized. Some researchers, in fact, have found that 42 percent of men whose partners were admitted to a psychiatric mother-baby unit met the *DSM-IV-TR* criteria for major depression. Just driving to the hospital knowing that one's partner will be receiving psychiatric treatment can be extremely stressful. And psychiatric units are not pretty places. Seeing the mother of one's child locked up in one can be a severely traumatic experience; in addition, those patients who are most seriously ill will probably be on high doses of medication that cause them to appear zombie-like. The whole experience, in short, turns an event that was meant to be full of joy into a nightmarish interlude rife with fear, frustration, and humiliation. And if the woman doesn't consent to treatment and has to be held against her will, her partner may also feel guilty and conflicted.

Family and friends who don't truly understand the situation may oppose hospitalization, inadvertently sabotage the treatment, and even blame the woman's partner for her situation. I've heard people suggest yoga or herbal treatments for women who were experiencing full-blown psychosis, and I've heard of men who were criticized for "punishing" their partners because they were ill. In light of all this, all I can do is to reassure the partners of these patients that they are safe, they are being well cared for, and they do really need to be there.

For the man who is himself emotionally unstable, however, coping with a partner's depression may be more than he can deal with on his own. The husband of one of my patients actually begged me to hospitalize his wife, even though I didn't think she was sick enough to require it, because, he said, if I didn't he would surely collapse. What I did in that instance was to have the woman's mother come to see her through her recovery and also to refer the husband to a colleague for treatment of his own depression.

When both partners are depressed, the concern, of course, is what effect the parents' depression will have on the baby and other members of the family. Even in the best of circumstances the birth of a baby alters the dynamics of the family as a whole and requires all members of the unit to reorganize and adjust. When the mother is coping with postpartum depression, the adjustment becomes that much harder for everyone. And if both parents are depressed, the problem can seem almost insurmountable. In that situation, I always recommend that both parents seek help immediately and that they find a trustworthy caregiver to look after the baby because it is virtually impossible to nurture an infant properly when one is in a depressed state.

Whatever the circumstances, however, the one thing both parents must always bear in mind is that depression is an illness and not anybody's fault, that it is treatable, and that they must be supportive of each other, both for their own sakes and for the sake of their newborn child.

EPILOGUE

Writing this book has been such a priority that I can only compare its significance and my devotion to completing it to the birth of my own children. I have breathed it, I have slept with it, I have loved it, and it has been worth it.

As I write these final pages I am filled with both elation and relief. I've come to the end of a long journey that began at a conference in Berlin almost three years ago. In the audience, as it turned out, was a health reporter for *Elle* magazine who called when I returned home to tell me that she wanted to write an article about the work I was doing in order to get this important and potentially life-transforming information to as many women as possible. At the end of our conversation she said, "You know, Shaila, you're going to write a book that will reach a much wider audience than even I can in the magazine; it's going to touch the hearts and minds of millions of women, and it's long overdue!" I promised her then that I would write that book, and now I've fulfilled my promise.

I wrote the first words on beautiful Vancouver Island, where I was scheduled to give a talk on the use of medication in pregnancy the next day. It was a blustery night, and as I sat on the balcony of my hotel room looking out over the ocean, it seemed to me that the stormy sea somehow symbolized the emotional ups and downs of women's moods. The following day dawned bright and sunny; the storm had passed and the sea was once more calm. Again, as I sipped my morning tea, I was struck by the similarity between the calmness of the ocean after the passing of a storm and the leveling out of mood that occurs when the emotional storm of depression subsides.

I know that when my patients are in the midst of a storm of emotions, they need to believe and trust that those stormy feelings will pass. So whenever I see a new patient, the first thing I do is to assure her that she *is* going to get better, that she is going to love her baby, and yes, she is going to be a great mother. Soon, I tell her, her negative thoughts will pass, her sleepless nights and her nightmares will end; it is just a matter of time. Being able to give her that assurance is, to me, the most important part of my job.

This book, then, has been about hope. And my hope is that any woman who is depressed and who has read this far will be feeling empowered to challenge the stereotypical beliefs of her health care providers and insist upon getting the help she needs and deserves. I hope it will open the eyes of millions of people and validate the feelings of every woman who sees herself reflected in my patients' stories.

It was in the eleventh century that Trotula of Salerno wrote about the suffering women experienced with relation to childbirth, and ten centuries later, although we are still struggling to convince health care providers of the association between pregnancy and mental illness, we are finally making significant progress. We have yet to find a treatment that is perfect, but the very fact that depressed and anxious women are receiving attention is a tremendous step forward. Over the next few years, through research, an even better understanding of complicated brain chemistry, and the development of newer, safer medications, as well as sophisticated psychotherapies, the picture will become that much brighter and the suffering less.

In 1979, at the start of my career, I could never have imagined that I would see the day when women with serious mental illness were cared for in a hospital while their babies were being looked after in the nursery next door. The past twenty-five years have been incredible, and I look forward to an even more amazing twenty-five to come.

*   *   *

I have tried my very best to be as honest with you, my readers, as I am with my patients. Most times my patients appreciate this and feel that they can trust me. I hope that you now feel you can trust me as well.

To cement that trust, I would like to end on a very personal note. As I complete this writing I am preparing to leave for India, where my mother, Mandakini, and I will celebrate her seventy-fifth birthday together in the city of Mumbai.

When my father died in 1992, my mother lost her companion of forty-five years, her best friend, and the father of her three children. When she came to visit me in Vancouver a year later, I hardly recognized the woman who greeted me at the airport. She had gone from a beautiful, outgoing, vivacious, colorful woman to a dark, lifeless, joyless person, dressed all in gray, drained of energy, and filled with negativity, anger, and bitterness. When I finally spotted her, sitting in a corner with her suitcase like a lost, frightened child, I immediately thought of my patient Corrine, a thirty-four-year-old artist whose family was initially alerted to her depressed state when they noticed that the bleak blacks and grays of her paintings were nothing like the yellows, reds, and greens she normally used in her work. To escape the dreariness of February in Vancouver, I took my mother for a holiday to Hawaii. One evening, as we were sitting on the beach of the beautiful Royal Hawaiian Hotel in Honolulu and enjoying the sunset, my mother suddenly turned to me and said, "Shaila, I am choking and I think I am just going to die." And with that she burst into a frenzy of tears.

Thirteen years have passed now since that trip to Honolulu, and my mother is a changed person. She continues to take the Zoloft without which she would not survive, and—again like Corinne, who after treatment resumed painting in the bright yellows and oranges that reflected the vibrancy that had returned to her life—my mother is once more living a wonderfully rich life.

Sometimes when I lecture in India, she stands up with me at the front of the room and tells the audience, many of whom still cannot understand, what depression is really about. She talks about it with her relatives and neighbors, spreading the word that I have tried to spread in North America. My mother is my messenger to the women of India, and I am proud of her openness and honesty, especially because she comes from a time when mental illness carried a terrible stigma and a cultural background in which openly discussing such personal problems would have been virtually unthinkable.

I say to my mother bravo, which is what I say to any woman who is brave enough to find a way through her personal darkness to the light that I know will shine on her once more.

RESOURCES

Antiepileptic Drug Pregnancy Registry
888-233-2334
www.aedpregnancyregistry.org (anticonvulsant exposure)
www.moodpreg.org (specifically for mood disorders and pregnancy)
Information also available on neurodevelopmental follow-up studies

BC Reproductive Mental Health Program
www.bcrmh.com; www.bcwomens.ca

Bupropion Pregnancy Registry (GlaxoSmithKline)
800-336-2176

Center for Women's Mental Health
(Massachusetts General Hospital, Boston, MA)
www.womensmentalhealth.org

Depression
www.depression-net.com

Dr. Shaila Misri
www.wellmother.com

Emory Women's Mental Health Program (Emory University, Atlanta, GA)
www.emorywomensprogram.org

Lamotrigine Pregnancy Registry (GlaxoSmithKline)
800-336-2176

Micromedex
800-525-9083
email: *mdx.info@tomson.com*

Motherisk Program at Sick Children's Hospital, Toronto
www.motherisk.org

Postpartum Depression
www.postpartum.org

Postpartum Support International
http://www.postpartum.net

ReproTox
202-293-5237
www.reprotox.org

TERIS
206-543-2465
www.depts.washington.edu/~terisweb
Encompasses ReproTox, TERIS, ReproRisk, and other databases

APPENDIX:

DIAGNOSTIC TOOLS FOR DEPRESSION

EDINBURGH POSTNATAL DEPRESSION SCALE (EPDS)
J.L. Cox, J.M. Holden, R. Sagovsky. Department of Psychiatry, University of Edinburgh

As you have recently had a baby, we would like to know how you are feeling. Please mark the answer which comes closest to how you have felt IN THE PAST 7 DAYS, not just how you feel today.

Here is an example, already completed.
I have felt happy:
- ☐ Yes, all the time
- ☒ Yes, most of the time
- ☐ No, not very often
- ☐ No, not at all

This would mean "I have felt happy most of the time" during the past week.
Please complete the other questions the same way.

In the past 7 days:

1. I have been able to laugh and see the funny side of things
   - ☐ As much as I always could   0
   - ☐ Not quite so much now   1
   - ☐ Definitely not so much now   2
   - ☐ Not at all   3

253

In the past 7 days:

2. I have looked forward with enjoyment to things

☐ As much as I ever did   0
☐ Rather less than I used to   1
☐ Definitely less than I used to   2
☐ Hardly at all   3

3. I have blamed myself unnecessarily when things went wrong

☐ Yes, most of the time   3
☐ Yes, some of the time   2
☐ Not very often   1
☐ No, never   0

4. I have been anxious or worried for no good reason

☐ No, not at all   0
☐ Hardly ever   1
☐ Yes, sometimes   2
☐ Yes, very often   3

5. I have felt scared or panicky for no very good reason

☐ Yes, quite a lot   3
☐ Yes, sometimes   2
☐ No, not much   1
☐ No, not at all   0

6. Things have been getting on top of me

☐ Yes, most of the time I haven't been able to cope   3
☐ Yes, sometimes I haven't been coping as well as usual   2
☐ No, most of the time I have coped quite well   1
☐ No, I have been coping as well as ever   0

7. I have been so unhappy that I have had difficulty sleeping

☐ Yes, most of the time   3
☐ Yes, sometimes   2
☐ Not very often   1
☐ No, not at all   0

8. I have felt sad or miserable

☐ Yes, most of the time   3
☐ Yes, quite often   2
☐ Not very often   1
☐ No, not at all   0

9. I have been so unhappy that I have been crying

    ☐ Yes, most of the time   3

    ☐ Yes, quite often   2

    ☐ Only occasionally   1

    ☐ No, never   0

10. The thought of harming myself has occurred to me

    ☐ Yes, quite often   3

    ☐ Sometimes   2

    ☐ Hardly ever   1

    ☐ Never   0

A score of 12 or above indicates postnatal depression.

Translations of the scale, and guidance as to its use, may be found in Cox, J.L. & Holden, J. (2003), *Perinatal Mental Health: A Guide to the Edinburgh Postnatal Depression Scale.* London: Gaskell.

ANTENATAL RISK QUESTIONNAIRE

PLEASE COMPLETE ALL ITEMS

Please circle numbers 1–5 or check Yes/No, as applicable

1. When you were growing up, did you feel your mother was emotionally supportive of you? (If you had no mother circle 6).

1	2	3	4	5	6
VERY MUCH		SOMEWHAT		NOT AT ALL	

2. Before this pregnancy did you ever have a period of 2 weeks or more when you felt particularly miserable or depressed? If so, did this

   a) seriously interfere with your work and your relationships with friends and family?

1	2	3	4	5
NOT AT ALL		SOMEWHAT		VERY MUCH

   b) lead you to seek professional help?   Yes ☐   No ☐
   Did you see a Psychiatrist ☐   Psychologist/Counsellor ☐

   _____

   (Name of professional)

   c) Did you take tablets/herbal medicine? No ☐ Yes ☐ Please specify

   _____

3. Is your relationship with your partner an emotionally supportive one? (If you have no partner circle 6)

1	2	3	4	5	6
VERY MUCH		SOMEWHAT		NOT AT ALL	

4. Have you had any major stresses, changes or losses in the last 12 months (e.g. separation, moving house, domestic violence, unemployment, bereavement)?   Yes ☐   No ☐

   a) If so please list these:_____

   _____

   b) Were you distressed by these stresses, changes or losses?

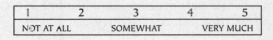

1	2	3	4	5
NOT AT ALL		SOMEWHAT		VERY MUCH

5. Would you generally consider yourself a worrier?

1	2	3	4	5
NOT AT ALL		SOMEWHAT		VERY MUCH

6. In general, do you become upset if you do not have order in your life (e.g. regular timetable, a tidy house)?

1	2	3	4	5
NOT AT ALL		SOMEWHAT		VERY MUCH

7. Do you feel you will have people you can depend on for emotional support when you go home with your baby?

1	2	3	4	5
NOT AT ALL		SOMEWHAT		VERY MUCH

8. Were you emotionally abused when you were growing up?

Yes ☐   No ☐

9. Have you ever been sexually or physically abused?

Yes ☐   No ☐

ANTENATAL PSYCHOSOCIAL HEALTH ASSESSMENT (ALPHA)

Antenatal psychosocial problems may be associated with unfavorable post-partum outcomes. The questions on this form are suggested ways of inquiring about psychosocial health.

Issues of **high** concern to the woman, her family or the caregiver usually indicate a need for additional supports or services. When **some** concerns are identified, follow-up and/or referral should be considered. Additional information can be obtained from the ALPHA Guide.*

Please consider the sensitivity of this information before sharing it with other caregivers.

ANTENATAL FACTORS	CONCERN	COMMENTS/PLAN
FAMILY FACTORS **Social support (*CA, WA*, PD)** • How does your partner/family feel about your pregnancy? • Who will be helping you when you go home with your baby?	☐ Low ☐ Some ☐ High	
Recent stressful life events (*CA, WA, PD*, PI) • What life changes have you experienced this year? • What changes are you planning during this pregnancy?	☐ Low ☐ Some ☐ High	
Couple's relationship (*CD, PD*, WA, CA) • How would you describe your relationship with your partner? • What do you think your relationship will be like after the birth?	☐ Low ☐ Some ☐ High	

ASSOCIATED POSTPARTUM OUTCOMES

The antenatal factors in the left column have been shown to be associated with the postpartum outcomes listed below. *Bold, Italics* indicates *good* evidence of association. Regular text indicates fair evidence of association.

CA - Child Abuse   CD - Couple Dysfunction   PI - Physical Illness

PD - Postpartum Depression   WA - Woman Abuse

ANTENATAL FACTORS	CONCERN	COMMENTS/PLAN
MATERNAL FACTORS		
Prenatal care (late onset) *(WA)* • First prenatal visit in third trimester? (check records)	☐ Low ☐ Some ☐ High	
Prenatal education (refusal or quit) *(CA)* • What are your plans for prenatal classes?	☐ Low ☐ Some ☐ High	
Feelings toward pregnancy after 20 weeks *(CA, WA)* • How did you feel when you just found out you were pregnant? • How do you feel about it now?	☐ Low ☐ Some ☐ High	
Relationship with parents in childhood *(CA)* • How did you get along with your parents? • Did you feel loved by your parents?	☐ Low ☐ Some ☐ High	
Self-esteem *(CA,* WA) • What concerns do you have about becoming/being a mother?	☐ Low ☐ Some ☐ High	
History of psychiatric/emotional problems *(CA,* WA, PD) • Have you ever had emotional problems? • Have you ever seen a psychiatrist or therapist?	☐ Low ☐ Some ☐ High	
Depression in this pregnancy *(PD)* • How has your mood been during this pregnancy?	☐ Low ☐ Some ☐ High	
SUBSTANCE USE **Alcohol/drug abuse** (WA, CA) (1 drink = 1 ½ oz liquor, 12 oz beer, 5 oz wine) • How many drinks of alcohol do you have per week? • Are there times when you drink more than that? • Do you or your partner use recreational drugs? • Do you or your partner have a problem with alcohol or drugs? • Consider CAGE (Cut down, Annoyed, Guilty, Eye opener)	☐ Low ☐ Some ☐ High	

ANTENATAL FACTORS	CONCERN	COMMENTS/PLAN
FAMILY VIOLENCE **Woman or partner experienced or witnessed abuse (physical, emotional, sexual) (CA, WA)** • What was your parents' relationship like? • Did your father ever scare or hurt your mother? • Did your parents ever scare or hurt you? • Were you ever sexually abused as a child?	☐ Low ☐ Some ☐ High	
Current or past woman abuse (WA, CA, PD) • How do you and your partner solve arguments? • Do you ever feel frightened by what your partner says or does? • Have you ever been hit/pushed/slapped by a partner? • Has your partner ever humiliated you or psychologically abused you in other ways? • Have you ever been forced to have sex against your will?	☐ Low ☐ Some ☐ High	
Previous child abuse by woman or partner (CA) • Do you/your partner have children not living with you? If so, why? • Have you ever had involvement with a child protection agency (i.e., Children's Aid Society)?	☐ Low ☐ Some ☐ High	
Child discipline (CA) • How were you disciplined as a child? • How do you think you will discipline your child? • How do you deal with your kids at home when they misbehave?	☐ Low ☐ Some ☐ High	

FOLLOW-UP PLAN:
☐ Supportive counseling by provider
☐ Additional prenatal appointments
☐ Additional postpartum appointments
☐ Additional well-baby visits
☐ Public Health referral
☐ Prenatal education services

FOLLOW UP PLAN cont'd:

☐ Nutritionist
☐ Community resources / mothers' group
☐ Homecare
☐ Parenting classes / parents' support group
☐ Addiction treatment programs
☐ Smoking cessation resources
☐ Social Worker
☐ Psychologist / Psychiatrist
☐ Psychotherapist / marital / family therapist
☐ Assaulted women's helpline / shelter / counseling
☐ Legal advice
☐ Children's Aid Society
☐ Other: _____
☐ Other: _____
☐ Other: _____
☐ Other: _____

COMMENTS:

_____
_____
_____

POSTPARTUM DEPRESSION PREDICTORS INVENTORY (PDPI)—
REVISED AND GUIDE QUESTIONS FOR ITS USE

During Pregnancy   **Check One**

Marital status
1. Single   ☐
2. Married/cohabitating   ☐
3. Separated   ☐
4. Divorced   ☐
5. Widowed   ☐
6. Partnered   ☐

Socioeconomic status
  Low   ☐
  Middle   ☐
  High   ☐

Self-esteem	Yes	No
Do you feel good about yourself as a person?	☐	☐
Do you feel worthwhile?	☐	☐
Do you feel you have a number of good qualities as a person?	☐	☐

Prenatal depression
1. Have you felt depressed during your pregnancy?   ☐   ☐
  If yes, when and how long have you been feeling
    this way?
  If yes, how mild or severe would you consider your
    depression?

Prenatal anxiety
  Have you been feeling anxious during your pregnancy?   ☐   ☐
  If yes, how long have you been feeling this way?

Unplanned/unwanted pregnancy
  Was the pregnancy planned?   ☐   ☐
  Is the pregnancy unwanted?   ☐   ☐

History of previous depression
1. Before this pregnancy, have you ever been depressed?   ☐   ☐
  If yes, when did you experience this depression?
  If yes, have you been under a physician's care
    for this past depression?   ☐   ☐
  If yes, did the physician prescribe any medication for
    your depression?   ☐   ☐

During Pregnancy	Check One	

Social support

	Yes	No
1. Do you feel you receive adequate emotional support from your partner?	☐	☐
2. Do you feel you receive adequate instrumental support from your partner (e.g., help with household chores or babysitting)?	☐	☐
3. Do you feel you can rely on your partner when you need help?	☐	☐
4. Do you feel you can confide in your partner?	☐	☐
(repeat same questions for family and again for friends)		

Marital satisfaction

1. Are you satisfied with your marriage (or living arrangement)?	☐	☐
2. Are you currently experiencing any marital problems?	☐	☐
3. Are things going well between you and your partner?	☐	☐

Life stress

1. Are you currently experiencing any stressful events in your life such as:

financial problems	☐	☐
marital problems	☐	☐
death in the family	☐	☐
serious illness in the family	☐	☐
moving	☐	☐
unemployment	☐	☐
job change	☐	☐

After delivery, add the following items

Child care stress

1. Is your infant experiencing any health problems?	☐	☐
2. Are you having problems with your baby feeding?	☐	☐
3. Are you having problems with your baby sleeping?	☐	☐

Infant temperament

1. Would you consider your baby irritable or fussy?	☐	☐
2. Does your baby cry a lot?	☐	☐
3. Is your baby difficult to console or soothe?	☐	☐

Maternity blues

1. Did you experience a brief period of tearfulness and mood swings during the 1st week after delivery?	☐	☐

Beck, Cheryl. Revision of Postpartum Depression Predictors Inventory. *JOGNN* 2002; 31(4):394–402.

REFERENCES

Chapter 1

Barnard A, Spencer J, eds. *Encyclopedia of social and cultural anthropology*. New York: Routledge, 1996.

Kitzinger S. *Ourselves as mothers*. Reading, MA: Addison-Wesley, 1994.

Chapter 2

American Psychiatric Association. *Diagnostic and statistical manual of mental disorders, 4th ed., text revision (DSM-IV-TR)*. Washington, D.C.: American Psychiatric Association, 2000.

Bhatia SC, Bhatia SK. Depression in women: diagnostic and treatment considerations. *American Family Physicians*. 1999;60(1):225–34.

Burt VK, Stein K. Epidemiology of depression throughout the female life cycle. *J Clin Psychiatry*. 2002;63 Suppl 7:9–15.

Campagne DM. Screening depressive patients in pregnancy with the pregnancy mood profile. *J Reprod Med*. 2003;48(10):813–7.

Cohen LS. Gender-specific considerations in the treatment of mood disorders in women across the life cycle. *J Clin Psychiatry*. 2003;64 Suppl 15:18–29.

Desai HD, Jann MW. Major depression in women: a review of the literature. *J Am Pharm Assoc (Wash)*. 2000;40(4):525–37.

Kelly R. Depression in women across the reproductive life cycle. *NAMI California*. 1999;10(4):16–18.

Kessler RC, McGonagle KA, Swartz M, et al. Sex and depression in the National Comorbidity Survey, 1: lifetime prevalence, chronicity and recurrence. *J Affect Disord.* 1993;29:85–96.

Magnusson A, Boivin D. Seasonal affective disorder: an overview. *Chronobiol Int.* 2003;20(2):189–207.

Murray CJL, Lopez ED, eds. *A comprehensive assessment of mortality and disability from diseases, injuries, and risk factors in 1990 and projected to 2020.* The Global Burden of Disease and Injury Series, vol 1. Cambridge, MA: Harvard University Press, 1996.

Ross LE, Steiner M. A biopsychosocial approach to premenstrual dysphoric disorder. *Psychiatr Clin North Am.* 2003;26(3):529–46.

Yonkers KA. Special issues related to the treatment of depression in women. *J Clin Psychiatry.* 2003;64 Suppl 18:8–13.

Yonkers KA, Pearlstein T, Rosenheck RA. Premenstrual disorders: bridging research and clinical reality. *Arch Women Ment Health.* 2003;6(4):287–92.

Chapter 3

Buckwalter JG, Stanczyk FZ, McCleary CA, Bluestein BW, Buckwalter DK, Rankin KP, Chang L, Goodwin TM. Pregnancy, the postpartum, and steroid hormones: effects on cognition and mood. *Psychoneuroendocrinology.* 1999;24(1):69–84.

Gregoire AJ, Kumar R, Everitt B, Henderson AF, Studd JW. Transdermal oestrogen for treatment of severe postnatal depression. *Lancet.* 1996;347 (9006):930–3.

Hohlagschwandtner M, Husslein P, Klier C, Ulm B. Correlation between serum testosterone levels and peripartal mood states. *Acta Obstet Gynecol Scand.* 2001;80(4):326–30.

Pearson Murphy BE, Steinberg SI, Hu FY, Allison CM. Neuroactive ring A-reduced metabolites of progesterone in human plasma during pregnancy: elevated levels of 5 alpha-dihydroprogesterone in depressed patients during the latter half of pregnancy. *J Clin Endocrinol Metab.* 2001;86(12):5981–7.

Sichel DA, Cohen LS, Robertson LM, Ruttenberg A, Rosenbaum JF. Prophylactic estrogen in recurrent postpartum affective disorder. *Biol Psychiatry.* 1995;38(12):814–8.

Chapter 4

Altshuler LL, Hendrick V, Cohen LS. Course of mood and anxiety disorders during pregnancy and the postpartum period. *J Clin Psychiatry.* 1998;59 Suppl 2:29–33.

Andersson L, Sundström-Poromaa I, Bixo M, Wulff M, Bondestam K, Åström M. Point prevalence of psychiatric disorders during the second trimester of pregnancy: a population-based study. *Am J Obstet Gynecol.* 2003;189(1): 148–54.

Atkinson AK, Rickel AU. Postpartum depression in primiparous parents. *J Abnorm Psychol.* 1984;93(1):115–9.

Bennett HA, Einarson A, Taddio A, Koren G, Einarson TR. Prevalence of depression during pregnancy: systematic review. *Obstet Gynecol.* 2004;103(4): 698–709.

Cox JL, Connor Y, Kendell RE. Prospective study of the psychiatric disorders of childbirth. *Br J Psychiatry.* 1982;140:111–7.

Einarson A, Selby P, Koren G. Abrupt discontinuation of psychotropic drugs during pregnancy: fear of teratogenic risk and impact of counselling. *J Psychiatry Neurosci.* 2001;26(1):44–8.

Evans J, Heron J, Francomb H, Oke S, Golding J. Cohort study of depressed mood during pregnancy and after childbirth. *BMJ.* 2001;323(7307):257–60.

Gotlib IH, Whiffen VE, Mount JH, Milne K, Cordy NI. Prevalence rates and demographic characteristics associated with depression in pregnancy and the postpartum. *J Consult Clin Psychol.* 1989;57(2):269–74.

Heilemann M, Frutos L, Lee K, Kury FS. Protective strength factors, resources, and risks in relation to depressive symptoms among childbearing women of Mexican descent. *Health Care Women Int.* 2004;25(1):88–106.

Hendrick V, Altshuler L. Management of major depression during pregnancy. *Am J Psychiatry.* 2002;159(10):1667–73.

Hendrick V, Altshuler L, Cohen L, Stowe Z. Evaluation of mental health and depression during pregnancy: position paper. *Psychopharmacol Bull.* 1998; 34(3):297–9.

Josefsson A, Berg G, Nordin C, Sydsjo G. Prevalence of depressive symptoms in late pregnancy and postpartum. *Acta Obstet Gynecol Scand.* 2001; 80(3):251–5.

Klein M, Essex MJ. Pregnant or depressed? The effect of overlap between symptoms of depression and somatic complaints of pregnancy on rates of major depression in the second trimester. *Depression.* 1995;2:308–14.

Llewellyn AM, Stowe ZN, Nemeroff CB. Depression during pregnancy and the puerperium. *J Clin Psychiatry.* 1997;58 Suppl 15:26–32.

McKee MD, Cunningham M, Jankowski KR, Zayas L. Health-related functional status in pregnancy: relationship to depression and social support in a multi-ethnic population. *Obstet Gynecol.* 2001;97(6):988–93.

Nonacs R, Cohen LS. Assessment and treatment of depression during pregnancy: an update. *Psychiatr Clin North Am.* 2003;26(3):547–62.

Small R, Lumley J, Yelland J. Cross-cultural experiences of maternal depression:

associations and contributing factors for Vietnamese, Turkish and Filipino immigrant women in Victoria, Australia. *Ethn Health*. 2003;8(3):189–206.

Zayas LH, Cunningham M, McKee MD, Jankowski KR. Depression and negative life events among pregnant African-American and Hispanic women. *Women's Health Issues*. 2002;12(1):16–22.

Chapter 5

Anderson KM, Sharpe M, Rattray A, Irvine DS. Distress and concerns in couples referred to a specialist infertility clinic. *J Psychosom Res*. 2003;54(4):353–5.

Berg BJ, Wilson JF. Psychiatric morbidity in the infertile population: a reconceptualization. *Fertil Steril*. 1990;53(4):654–61.

Beutel M, Deckardt R, von Rad M, Weiner H. Grief and depression after miscarriage: their separation, antecedents, and course. *Psychosom Med*. 1995; 57(6):517–26.

Dhaliwal LK, Gupta KR, Gopalan S, Kulhara P. Psychological aspects of infertility due to various causes—prospective study. *Int J Fertil Womens Med*. 2004;49(1):44–8.

Franche RL, Mikail SF. The impact of perinatal loss on adjustment to subsequent pregnancy. *Soc Sci Med*. 1999;48(11):1613–23.

Hunfeld JA, Taselaar-Kloos AK, Agterberg G, Wladimiroff JW, Passchier J. Trait anxiety, negative emotions, and the mothers' adaptation to an infant born subsequent to late pregnancy loss: a case-control study. *Prenat Diagn*. 1997;17(9):843–51.

Johanson R, Chapman G, Murray D, Johnson I, Cox J. The North Staffordshire Maternity Hospital prospective study of pregnancy-associated depression. *J Psychosom Obstet Gynaecol*. 2000;21(2):93–7.

Kee BS, Jung BJ, Lee SH. A study on psychological strain in IVF patients. *J Assist Reprod Genet*. 2000;17(8):445–8.

Klier CM, Geller PA, Ritsher JB. Affective disorders in the aftermath of miscarriage: a comprehensive review. *Arch Women Ment Health*. 2002;5(4):129–49.

Martin M. Infertility. In: DeCherney AH, Pernoll ML, eds. *Current obstetric and gynecologic diagnosis and treatment*, 8th ed. Norwalk, CT: Appleton & Lange, 1994.

Meller W, Burns LH, Crow S, Grambsch P. Major depression in unexplained infertility. *J Psychosom Obstet Gynaecol*. 2002;23(1):27–30.

Neugebauer R. Depressive symptoms at two months after miscarriage: interpreting study findings from an epidemiological versus clinical perspective. *Depress Anxiety*. 2003;17(3):152–61.

Rehner J. *Infertility: old myths, new meanings*. Toronto, ON: Second Story Press, 1989.

Stewart DE. Incidence of postpartum abuse in women with a history of abuse during pregnancy. CMAJ. 1994;151(11):1601–4.

Swanson KM. Predicting depressive symptoms after miscarriage: a path analysis based on the Lazarus paradigm. J Womens Health Gend Based Med. 2000;9(2):191–206.

Chapter 6

Katon W, Von Korff M, Lin E, Lipscomb P, Russo J, Wagner E, Polk E. Distressed high utilizers of medical care. DSM-III-R diagnoses and treatment needs. Gen Hosp Psychiatry. 1990;12(6):355–62.

Kelly RH, Russo J, Katon W. Somatic complaints among pregnant women cared for in obstetrics: normal pregnancy or depressive and anxiety symptom amplification revisited? Gen Hosp Psychiatry. 2001;23(3):107–13.

Sundström IM, Bixo M, Bjorn I, Åström M. Prevalence of psychiatric disorders in gynecologic outpatients. Am J Obstet Gynecol. 2001;184(2):8–13.

Chapter 7

Panic Disorder

Andersson L, Sundström-Poromaa I, Bixo M, Wulff M, Bondestam K, Åström M. Point prevalence of psychiatric disorders during the second trimester of pregnancy: a population-based study. Am J Obstet Gynecol. 2003;189 (1):148–54.

Andersson L, Sundström-Poromaa I, Wulff M, Åström M, Bixo M. Neonatal outcome following maternal antenatal depression and anxiety: a population-based study. Am J Epidemicl. 2004;159(9):872–81.

Cohen LS, Sichel DA, Dimmock JA, Rosenbaum JF. Impact of pregnancy on panic disorder: a case series. J Clin Psychiatry. 1994;55(7):284–8.

Cohen LS, Sichel DA, Dimmock JA, Rosenbaum JF. Postpartum course in women with preexisting panic disorder. J Clin Psychiatry. 1994;55(7):289–92.

Fraiberg S, Adelson E, Shapiro V. Ghosts in the nursery. A psychoanalytic approach to the problems of impaired infant-mother relationships. J Am Acad Child Psychiatry. 1975;14(3):387–421.

George DT, Ladenheim JA, Nutt DJ. Effect of pregnancy on panic attacks. Am J Psychiatry. 1987;144(8):1078–9.

Grote NK, Frank E. Difficult-to-treat depression: the role of contexts and co-morbidities. Biol Psychiatry. 2003;53(8):660–70.

Halbreich U. Anxiety disorders in women: a developmental and lifecycle perspective. Depress Anxiety. 2003;17(3):107–10.

Heron J, O'Connor TG, Evans J, Golding J, Glover V. The course of anxiety and depression through pregnancy and the postpartum in a community sample. *J Affect Disord.* 2004;80(1):65–73.

Kessler RC, Berglund P, Demler O, Jin R, Koretz D, Merikangas KR, Rush AJ, Walters EE, Wang PS. The epidemiology of major depressive disorder: results from the National Comorbidity Survey Replication (NCS-R). *JAMA.* 2003;289(23):3095–105.

Levine RE, Oandasan AP, Primeau LA, Berenson AB. Anxiety disorders during pregnancy and postpartum. *Am J Perinatol.* 2003;20(5):239–48.

Northcott CJ, Stein MB. Panic disorder in pregnancy. *J Clin Psychiatry.* 1994; 55(12):539–42.

Shear MK, Mammen O. Anxiety disorders in pregnant and postpartum women. *Psychopharmacol Bull.* 1995;31(4):693–703.

Weisberg RB, Paquette JA. Screening and treatment of anxiety disorders in pregnant and lactating women. *Womens Health Issues.* 2002;12(1):32–6.

Obsessive-Compulsive Disorder

Abramowitz J, Schwartz S, Moore K. Obsessional thoughts in postpartum females and their partners: content, severity and relationship with depression. *J Clin Psychol Med Set.* 2003;10(3):157–64.

Buttolph ML, Holland AD. Obsessive-compulsive disorders in pregnancy and childbirth. In: Jenike M, Baer L, Minichiello W, eds. *Obsessive-compulsive disorders: theory and management.* Pp. 89–97. Chicago: Year Book Medical, 1990.

Chelmow D, Halfin VP. Pregnancy complicated by obsessive-compulsive disorder. *J Matern Fetal Med.* 1997;6(1):31–4.

Hertzberg T, Leo RJ, Kim KY. Recurrent obsessive-compulsive disorder associated with pregnancy and childbirth. *Psychosomatics.* 1997;38(4): 386–8.

Ingram IM. Obsessional illness in mental hospital patients. *J Ment Sci.* 1961; 107:382–402.

Jennings KD, Ross S, Popper S, Elmore M. Thoughts of harming infants in depressed and nondepressed mothers. *J Affect Disord.* 1999;54(1–2):21–8.

Maina G, Albert U, Bogetto F, Vaschetto P, Ravizza L. Recent life events and obsessive-compulsive disorder (OCD): the role of pregnancy/delivery. *Psychiatry Research.* 1999;89:49–58.

Neziroglu F, Anemone R, Yaryura-Tobias JA. Onset of obsessive-compulsive disorder in pregnancy. *Am J Psychiatry.* 1992;149(7):947–50.

Sichel DA, Cohen LS, Dimmock JA, Rosenbaum JF. Postpartum obsessive compulsive disorder: a case series. *J Clin Psychiatry.* 1993;54(4):156–9.

Williams KE, Koran LM. Obsessive-compulsive disorder in pregnancy, the puerperium, and the premenstruum. *J Clin Psychiatry*. 1997;58(7):330–4; quiz 335–6.

Post-traumatic Stress Disorder

Loveland Cook CA, Flick LH, Homan SM, Campbell C, McSweeney M, Gallagher ME. Posttraumatic stress disorder in pregnancy: prevalence, risk factors, and treatment. *Obstet Gynecol*. 2004;103(4):710–7.

Moylan PL, Jones HE, Haug NA, Kissin WB, Svikis DS. Clinical and psychosocial characteristics of substance-dependent pregnant women with and without PTSD. *Addict Behav*. 2001;26(3):469–74.

Seng JS, Oakley DJ, Sampselle CM, Killion C, Graham-Bermann S, Liberzon I. Posttraumatic stress disorder and pregnancy complications. *Obstet Gynecol*. 2001;97(1):17–22.

Seng JS, Sparbel KJ, Low LK, Killion C. Abuse-related posttraumatic stress and desired maternity care practices: women's perspectives. *J Midwifery Womens Health*. 2002;47(5):360–70.

Soderquist J, Wijma K, Wijma B. Traumatic stress in late pregnancy. *J Anxiety Disord*. 2004;18(2):127–42.

Eating Disorders

Brinch M, Isager T, Tolstrup K. Anorexia nervosa and motherhood: reproduction pattern and mothering behavior of 50 women. *Acta Psychiatr Scand*. 1988;77(5):611–7.

Conrad R, Schablewski J, Schilling G, Liedtke R. Worsening of symptoms of bulimia nervosa during pregnancy. *Psychosomatics*. 2003;44(1):76–8.

Franko DL, Blais MA, Becker AE, Delinsky SS, Greenwood DN, Flores AT, Ekeblad ER, Eddy KT, Herzog DB. Pregnancy complications and neonatal outcomes in women with eating disorders. *Am J Psychiatry*. 2001;158(9): 1461–6.

Mitchell J, Seim H, Glotter D, Soll E, Pyle R. A retrospective study of pregnancy in bulimia nervosa. *Int J Eat Disord*. 1991;10:209–14.

Mitchell-Gieleghem A, Mittelstaedt ME, Bulik CM. Eating disorders and childbearing: concealment and consequences. *Birth*. 2002;29(3):182–91.

Bipolar Disorder

Ahokas A, Aito M, Rimon R. Positive treatment effect of estradiol in postpartum psychosis: a pilot study. *J Clin Psychiatry*. 2000;61(3):166–9.

Akdeniz F, Vahip S, Pirildar S, Vahip I, Doganer I, Bulut I. Risk factors associated with childbearing-related episodes in women with bipolar disorder. *Psychopathology*. 2003;36(5):234–8.

Blehar MC, DePaulo JR, Jr., Gershon ES, Reich T, Simpson SG, Nurnberger JI Jr. Women with bipolar disorder: findings from the NIMH Genetics Initiative sample. *Psychopharmacol Bull.* 1998;34(3):239–43.

Chaudron LH, Pies RW. The relationship between postpartum psychosis and bipolar disorder: a review. *J Clin Psychiatry.* 2003;64(11):1284–92.

Cohen LS, Sichel DA, Robertson LM, Heckscher E, Rosenbaum JF. Postpartum prophylaxis for women with bipolar disorder. *Am J Psychiatry.* 1995; 152(11):1641–5.

Freeman MP, Smith KW, Freeman SA, McElroy SL, Kmetz GE, Wright R, Keck PE Jr. The impact of reproductive events on the course of bipolar disorder in women. *J Clin Psychiatry.* 2002;63(4):284–7.

Grof P, Robbins W, Alda M, Berghoefer A, Vojtechovsky M, Nilsson A, Robertson C. Protective effect of pregnancy in women with lithium-responsive bipolar disorder. *J Affect Disord.* 2000;61(1–2):31–39.

Hansen HV, Andersen HS. Psychosis and pregnancy: five cases of severely ill women. *Nord J Psychiatry.* 2001;55(6):433–7.

Jones I, Craddock N. Familiality of the puerperal trigger in bipolar disorder: results of a family study. *Am J Psychiatry.* 2001;158(6):913–7.

Viguera AC, Cohen LS, Bouffard S, Whitfield TH, Baldessarini RJ. Reproductive decisions by women with bipolar disorder after prepregnancy psychiatric consultation. *Am J Psychiatry.* 2002;159(12):2102–4.

Viguera AC, Cohen LJ, Tondo L, Baldessarini RJ. Protective effect of pregnancy on the course of lithium-responsive bipolar I disorder. *J Affect Disord.* 2002;72(1):107–8; author reply 103–5.

Viguera AC, Nonacs R, Cohen LS, Tondo L, Murray A, Baldessarini RJ. Risk of recurrence of bipolar disorder in pregnant and nonpregnant women after discontinuing lithium maintenance. *Am J Psychiatry.* 2000;157(2):179–84.

Chapter 8

Abebe-Campino G, Offer D, Stahl B, Merlob P. Cardiac arrhythmia in a newborn infant associated with fluoxetine use during pregnancy. *Ann Pharmacother.* 2002;36:533–34.

Adab N, Jacoby A, Smith D, Chadwick D. Additional educational needs in children born to mothers with epilepsy. *J Neurol Neurosurg Psychiatry.* 2001;70(1):15–21.

Addis A, Dolovich LR, Einarson TR, Koren G. Can we use anxiolytics during pregnancy without anxiety? *Can Fam Physician.* 2000;46:549–51.

Addis A, Koren G. Safety of fluoxetine during the first trimester of pregnancy: a meta-analytical review of epidemiological studies. *Psychol Med.* 2000; 30(1):89–94.

Ahokas A, Aito M, Rimon R. Positive treatment effect of estradiol in post-partum psychosis: a pilot study. *J Clin Psychiatry*. 2000;61(3):166–9.

Ahokas A, Kaukoranta J, Aito M. Effect of oestradiol on postpartum depression. *Psychopharmacology (Berl)*. 1999;146(1):108–10.

Ahokas A, Kaukoranta J, Wahlbeck K, Aito M. Estrogen deficiency in severe postpartum depression: successful treatment with sublingual physiologic 17beta-estradiol: a preliminary study. *J Clin Psychiatry*. 2001;62(5): 332–6.

Altshuler LL, Cohen L, Szuba MP, Burt VK, Gitlin M, Mintz J. Pharmacologic management of psychiatric illness during pregnancy: dilemmas and guidelines. *Am J Psychiatry*. 1996;153(5):592–606.

Altshuler LL, Hendrick VC. Pregnancy and psychotropic medication: changes in blood levels. *J Clin Psychopharmacol*. 1996;16(1):78–80.

American Academy of Pediatrics. Use of psychoactive medication during pregnancy and possible effects on the fetus and newborn. Committee on Drugs. *Pediatrics*. 2000;105(4):880–7.

Baldwin JA, Davidson EJ, Pritchard AL, Ridings JE. The reproductive toxicology of paroxetine. *Acta Psychiatr Scand Suppl*. 1989;350:37–9.

Barki ZHK, Kravitz HM, Berki TM. Psychotropic medications in pregnancy. *Psychiatr Ann*. 1998;28:486–500.

Barnas C, Bergant A, Hummer M, Saria A, Fleischhacker WW. Clozapine concentrations in maternal and fetal plasma, amniotic fluid, and breast milk. *Am J Psychiatry*. 1994;151(6):945.

Bennett HA, Einarson A, Taddio A, Koren G, Einarson TR. Prevalence of depression during pregnancy: systematic review. *Obstet Gynecol*. 2004;103(4): 698–709.

Bergman U, Rosa FW, Baum C, Wiholm BE, Faich GA. Effects of exposure to benzodiazepine during fetal life. *Lancet*. 1992;340(8821):694–6.

Bescoby-Chambers N, Forster P, Bates G. Foetal valproate syndrome and autism: additional evidence of an association. *Dev Med Child Neurol*. 2001; 43(12):847.

Biswas PN, Wilton LV, Shakir SA. The pharmacovigilance of mirtazapine: results of a prescription event monitoring study on 13554 patients in England. *J Psychopharmacol*. 2003;17(1):121–6.

Blier P, Ward NM. Is there a role for 5-HT1A agonists in the treatment of depression? *Biol Psychiatry*. 2003;53(3):193–203.

Bloch M, Schmidt PJ, Danaceau M, Murphy J, Nieman L, Rubinow DR. Effects of gonadal steroids in women with a history of postpartum depression. *Am J Psychiatry*. 2000;157(6):924–30.

Boyer WF, Blumhardt CL. The safety profile of paroxetine. *J Clin Psychiatry*. 1992;53 Suppl:61–6.

Briggs G, Freeman R, Yaffe S. *Drugs in pregnancy and lactation*. Baltimore: Williams & Wilkins, 1998.

Brockington I. Postpartum psychiatric disorders. *Lancet*. 2004;363(9405): 303–10.

Chambers CD, Johnson KA, Dick LM, Felix RJ, Jones KL. Birth outcomes in pregnant women taking fluoxetine. *N Engl J Med*. 1996;335(14):1010–5.

Chang SI, McAuley JW. Pharmacotherapeutic issues for women of child-bearing age with epilepsy. *Ann Pharmacother*. 1998;32(7–8):794–801.

Cohen L, Altshuler L, Stowe Z, Faraone S. Reintroduction of antidepressant therapy across pregnancy in women who previously discontinued treatment: a preliminary retrospective study. *Psychother Psychosom*. 2004;73(6): 255–8.

Cohen LS, Friedman JM, Jefferson JW, Johnson EM, Weiner ML. A reevaluation of risk of in utero exposure to lithium. *JAMA*. 1994;271(2):146–50.

Cohen LS, Heller VL, Bailey JW, Grush L, Ablon JS, Bouffard SM. Birth outcomes following prenatal exposure to fluoxetine. *Biol Psychiatry*. 2000; 48(10):996–1000.

Cohen LS, Nonacs R, Viguera AC, Reminick A. Diagnosis and treatment of depression during pregnancy. *CNS Spectr*. 2004;9(3):209–16.

Cohen LS, Rosenbaum JF. Birth outcomes in pregnant women taking fluoxetine. *N Engl J Med*. 1997;336(12):872; author reply 873.

Cohen LS, Rosenbaum JF. Psychotropic drug use during pregnancy: weighing the risks. *J Clin Psychiatry*. 1998;59 Suppl 2:18–28.

Coleman FH, Christensen HD, Gonzalez CL, Rayburn WF. Behavioral changes in developing mice after prenatal exposure to paroxetine (Paxil). *Am J Obstet Gynecol*. 1999;181(5 Pt 1):1166–71.

Collins KO, Comer JB. Maternal haloperidol therapy associated with dyskinesia in a newborn. *Am J Health Syst Pharm*. 2003;60(21):2253–5.

Costei AM, Kozer E, Ho T, Ito S, Koren G. Perinatal outcome following third trimester exposure to paroxetine. *Arch Pediatr Adolesc Med*. 2002;156(11): 1129–32.

Craig M, Abel K. Drugs in pregnancy. Prescribing for psychiatric disorders in pregnancy and lactation. *Best Pract Res Clin Obstet Gynaecol*. 2001;15(6): 1013–30.

Currier GW, Simpson GM. Pregnancy and clozapine. *Psychiatr Serv*. 1998;49 (8):997.

Dean JC, Hailey H, Moore SJ, Lloyd DJ, Turnpenny PD, Little J. Long term health and neurodevelopment in children exposed to antiepileptic drugs before birth. *J Med Genet*. 2002;39(4):251–9.

Diav-Citrin O, Shechtman S, Arnon J, Ornoy A. Is carbamazepine teratogenic?

A prospective controlled study of 210 pregnancies. *Neurology.* 2001;57(2):321–4.

Dickson RA, Dawson DT. Olanzapine and pregnancy. *Can J Psychiatry.* 1998;43(2):196–7.

Doering PL, Stewart RB. The extent and character of drug consumption during pregnancy. *JAMA.* 1978;239(9):843–6.

Dolovich LR, Addis A, Vaillancourt JM, Power JD, Koren G, Einarson TR. Benzodiazepine use in pregnancy and major malformations or oral cleft: meta-analysis of cohort and case-control studies. *BMJ.* 1998;317(7162): 839–43.

Dominguez RA, Goodnick PJ. Adverse events after the abrupt discontinuation of paroxetine. *Pharmacotherapy.* 1995;15(6):778–80.

Edlund MJ, Craig TJ. Antipsychotic drug use and birth defects: an epidemiologic reassessment. *Compr Psychiatry.* 1984;25(1):32–7.

Edwards JG, Inman WH, Wilton L, Pearce GL. Prescription-event monitoring of 10,401 patients treated with fluvoxamine. *Br J Psychiatry.* 1994;164(3): 387–95.

Einarson A, Bonari L, Voyer-Lavigne S, Addis A, Matsui D, Johnson Y, Koren G. A multicentre prospective controlled study to determine the safety of trazodone and nefazodone use during pregnancy. *Can J Psychiatry.* 2003; 48(2):106–10.

Einarson A, Fatoye B, Sarkar M, Lavigne SV, Brochu J, Chambers C, Mastroiacovo P, Addis A, Matsui D, Schuler L, Einarson TR, Koren G. Pregnancy outcome following gestational exposure to venlafaxine: a multicenter prospective controlled study. *Am J Psychiatry.* 2001;158(10):1728–30.

Einarson A, Selby P, Koren G. Discontinuing antidepressants and benzodiazepines upon becoming pregnant. Beware of the risks of abrupt discontinuation. *Can Fam Physician.* 2001;47:489–90.

Einarson A, Selby P, Koren G. Abrupt discontinuation of psychotropic drugs during pregnancy: fear of teratogenic risk and impact of counselling. *J Psychiatry Neurosci.* 2001;26(1):44–8.

Epperson CN, Wisner KL, Yamamoto B. Gonadal steroids in the treatment of mood disorders. *Psychosom Med.* 1999;61(5):676–97.

Ericson A, Kallen B, Wiholm B. Delivery outcome after the use of antidepressants in early pregnancy. *Eur J Clin Pharmacol.* 1999;55(7):503–8.

Ernst CL, Goldberg JF. The reproductive safety profile of mood stabilizers, atypical antipsychotics, and broad-spectrum psychotropics. *J Clin Psychiatry.* 2002; 63 Suppl 4:42–55.

Evans J, Heron J, Francomb H, Oke S, Golding J. Cohort study of depressed mood during pregnancy and after childbirth. *BMJ.* 2001;323(7307):257–60.

Food and Drug Administration [Web site; updated 2004 June 9; cited 2004 Sept 23]. Summary minutes of the pediatrics subcommittee of the anti-infective drugs advisory committee. Available from: http://www.fda.gov/ohrms/dockets/ac/04/minutes/2004-4050M1.pdf.

Friedman EH. Neurobiology of behavioral changes after prenatal exposure to paroxetine (Paxil). *Am J Obstet Gynecol*. 2000;183(2):518–9.

Friedman J, Polifka J. *Teratogenic effects of drugs: a resource for clinicians (TERIS)*, 2nd ed. Baltimore, MD: John Hopkins University Press, 2000.

Gaily E, Kantola-Sorsa E, Hiilesmaa V, Isoaho M, Matila R, Kotila M, Nylund T, Bardy A, Kaaja E, Granstrom ML. Normal intelligence in children with prenatal exposure to carbamazepine. *Neurology*. 2004;62(1):28–32.

Gelenberg AJ. Citalopram (Celexa): SSRI #5. *Biol Ther Psychiatry Newsletter*. 1998:41–42.

Glaxo Wellcome Bupropion Pregnancy Registry Interim Report 9/1/97 to 2/28/03. Research Triangle Park, North Carolina, issued June 2003, pp. 1–22.

Gold LH. Psychopharmacologic treatment of depression during pregnancy. *Curr Womens Health Rep*. 2003;3(3):236–41.

Goldstein DJ. Effects of third trimester fluoxetine exposure on the newborn. *J Clin Psychopharmacol*. 1995;15(6):417–20.

Gorman JM. Medication and cognitive-behavioral therapy during pregnancy. *CNS Spectr*. 2004;9(3):170.

Gregoire AJ, Kumar R, Everitt B, Henderson AF, Studd JW. Transdermal oestrogen for treatment of severe postnatal depression. *Lancet*. 1996;347 (9006):930–3.

Grof P, Robbins W, Alda M, Berghoefer A, Vojtechovsky M, Nilsson A, Robertson C. Protective effect of pregnancy in women with lithium-responsive bipolar disorder. *J Affect Disord*. 2000;61(1–2):31–9.

Gupta S, Rangwani S. SSRIs in pregnancy. *J Fam Pract*. 1998;47(1):72.

Health Canada [Web site; updated 2004 Aug 17; cited 2004 Sept 23]. Health Canada advises of potential adverse effects of SSRIs and other anti-depressants on newborns. Available from: http://www.hc-sc.gc.ca/english/protection/warnings/2004/2004_44.htm.

Hendrick V, Smith LM, Suri R, Hwang S, Haynes D, Altshuler L. Birth outcomes after prenatal exposure to antidepressant medication. *Am J Obstet Gynecol*. 2003;188(3):812–5.

Hendrick V, Stowe ZN, Altshuler LL, Hostetter A, Fukuchi A. Paroxetine use during breast-feeding. *J Clin Psychopharmacol*. 2000;20(5):587–9.

Hendrick V, Stowe ZN, Altshuler LL, Hwang S, Lee E, Haynes D. Placental passage of antidepressant medications. *Am J Psychiatry*. 2003;160(5):993–6.

Heron J, O'Connor TG, Evans J, Golding J, Glover V. The course of anxiety and depression through pregnancy and the postpartum in a community sample. *J Affect Disord*. 2004;80(1):65–73.

Hiemke C, Hartter S. Pharmacokinetics of selective serotonin reuptake inhibitors. *Pharmacol Ther*. 2000;85(1):11–28.

Hoffbrand S, Howard L, Crawley H. Antidepressant drug treatment for postnatal depression. *Cochrane Database Syst Rev*. 2001(2):CD002018.

Hostetter A, Ritchie JC, Stowe ZN. Amniotic fluid and umbilical cord blood concentrations of antidepressants in three women. *Biol Psychiatry*. 2000; 48(10):1032–4.

Hostetter A, Stowe ZN, Strader JR Jr., McLaughlin E, Llewellyn A. Dose of selective serotonin uptake inhibitors across pregnancy: clinical implications. *Depress Anxiety*. 2000;11(2):51–7.

Howe AM, Oakes DJ, Woodman PD, Webster WS. Prothrombin and PIVKA-II levels in cord blood from newborn exposed to anticonvulsants during pregnancy. *Epilepsia*. 1999;40(7):980–4.

Iqbal MM. Prevention of neural tube defects by periconceptional use of folic acid. *Pediatr Rev*. 2000;21(2):58–66; quiz 66.

Iqbal MM, Gundlapalli SP, Ryan WG, Ryals T, Passman TE. Effects of antimanic mood-stabilizing drugs on fetuses, neonates, and nursing infants. *South Med J*. 2001;94(3):304–22.

Iqbal MM, Sobhan T, Aftab SR, Mahmud SZ. Diazepam use during pregnancy: a review of the literature. *Del Med J*. 2002;74(3):127–35.

Iqbal MM, Sobhan T, Mahmud SZ. The effects of lithium, valproic acid, and carbamazepine during pregnancy and lactation. *J Toxicol Clin Toxicol*. 2001;39(4):381–92.

Iqbal MM, Sobhan T, Ryals T. Effects of commonly used benzodiazepines on the fetus, the neonate, and the nursing infant. *Psychiatr Serv*. 2002;53(1):39–49.

Jacobson SJ, Jones K, Johnson K, Ceolin L, Kaur P, Sahn D, Donnenfeld AE, Rieder M, Santelli R, Smythe J, et al. Prospective multicentre study of pregnancy outcome after lithium exposure during first trimester. *Lancet*. 1992;339(8792):530–3.

Jeffries WS, Bochner F. The effect of pregnancy on drug pharmacokinetics. *Med J Aust*. 1988;149:675–7.

Jensen PN, Olesen OV, Bertelsen A, Linnet K. Citalopram and desmethylcitalopram concentrations in breast milk and in serum of mother and infant. *Ther Drug Monit*. 1997;19(2):236–9.

Jermain DM. Treatment of postpartum depression. *Am Pharm*. 1995;NS35(1):33–8, 45.

Joffe H, Cohen LS. Estrogen, serotonin, and mood disturbance: where is the therapeutic bridge? *Biol Psychiatry*. 1998;44(9):798–811.

Kallen B. Neonate characteristics after maternal use of antidepressants in late pregnancy. *Arch Pediatr Adolesc Med.* 2004;158(4):312–6.

Kaplan B, Modai I, Stoler M, Kitai E, Valevski A, Weizman A. Clozapine treatment and risk of unplanned pregnancy. *J Am Board Fam Pract.* 1995; 8:239–41.

Karuppaswamy J, Vlies R. The benefit of oestrogens and progestogens in postnatal depression. *J Obstet Gynaecol.* 2003;23(4):341–6.

Keller MB, Hirschfeld RM, Demyttenaere K, Baldwin DS. Optimizing outcomes in depression: focus on antidepressant compliance. *Int Clin Psychopharmacol.* 2002;17(6):265–71.

Kennedy D, Koren G. Valproic acid use in psychiatry: issues in treating women of reproductive age. *J Psychiatry Neurosci.* 1998;23(4):223–8.

Kent LS, Laidlaw JD. Suspected congenital sertraline dependence. *Br J Psychiatry.* 1995;167(3):412–3.

Kesim M, Yaris F, Kadioglu M, Yaris E, Kalyoncu NI, Ulku C. Mirtazapine use in two pregnant women: is it safe? *Teratology.* 2002;66:204.

Kim J, Riggs KW, Misri S, Kent N, Oberlander TF, Grunau RE, Fitzgerald C, Rurak DW. A comparison of fetal and neonatal exposure to paroxetine, sertraline and the R and S isomers of fluoxetine and norfluoxetine during pregnancy and breast-feeding. *Br J Clin Psychopharm.* Submitted.

Koren G. Discontinuation syndrome following late pregnancy exposure to antidepressants. *Arch Pediatr Adolesc Med.* 2004;158(4):307–8.

Koren G, Kennedy D. Safe use of valproic acid during pregnancy. *Can Fam Physician.* 1999;45:1451–3.

Koren G, Nulman I, Addis A. Outcome of children exposed in utero to fluoxetine: a critical review. *Depress Anxiety.* 1998;8 Suppl 1:27–31.

Kornstein SG, McEnany G. Enhancing pharmacologic effects in the treatment of depression in women. *J Clin Psychiatry.* 2000;61 Suppl 11:18–27.

Kulin NA, Pastuszak A, Sage SR, Schick-Boschetto B, Spivey G, Feldkamp M, Ormond K, Matsui D, Stein-Schechman AK, Cook L, Brochu J, Rieder M, Koren G. Pregnancy outcome following maternal use of the new selective serotonin reuptake inhibitors: a prospective controlled multicenter study. *JAMA.* 1998;279(8):609–10.

Laine K, Heikkinen T, Ekblad U, Kero P. Effects of exposure to selective serotonin reuptake inhibitors during pregnancy on serotonergic symptoms in newborns and cord blood monoamine and prolactin concentrations. *Arch Gen Psychiatry.* 2003;60(7):720–6.

Levine RE, Oandasan AP, Primeau LA, Berenson AB. Anxiety disorders during pregnancy and postpartum. *Am J Perinatol.* 2003;20(5):239–48.

Levy N, Smith MK. Lactation and psychotropic medications: treatment considerations. *Psychiatric Times.* 2000:62–65.

Lewis DP, Van Dyke DC, Stumbo PJ, Berg MJ. Drug and environmental factors associated with adverse pregnancy outcomes. Part I: antiepileptic drugs, contraceptives, smoking, and folate. *Ann Pharmacother*. 1998;32(7–8):802–17.

Littrell KH, Johnson CG, Peabody CD, Hilligoss N. Antipsychotics during pregnancy. *Am J Psychiatry*. 2000;157(8):1342.

Loebstein R, Koren G. Pregnancy outcome and neurodevelopment of children exposed in utero to psychoactive drugs: the Motherisk experience. *J Psychiatry Neurosci* 1997;22(3):192–6.

Malek-Ahmadi P. Olanzapine in pregnancy. *Ann Pharmacother*. 2001;35(10): 1294–5.

Malm H, Kajantie E, Kivirikko S, Kaariainen H, Peippo M, Somer M. Valproate embryopathy in three sets of siblings: further proof of hereditary susceptibility. *Neurology*. 2002;59(4):630–3.

Marano HE. Depression: beyond serotonin. *Psychology Today*. 1999;Mar-Apr:30.

Matalon S, Schechtman S, Goldzweig G, Ornoy A. The teratogenic effect of carbamazepine: a meta-analysis of 1255 exposures. *Reprod Toxicol*. 2002; 16(1):9–17.

Mattes JA. Fluoxetine and norfluoxetine. *Am J Psychiatry*. 1998;155(11):1637.

McElhatton PR, Garbis HM, Elefant E, Vial T, Bellemin B, Mastroiacovo P, Arnon J, Rodriguez-Pinilla E, Schaefer C, Pexieder T, Merlob P, Dal Verme S. The outcome of pregnancy in 689 women exposed to therapeutic doses of antidepressants. A collaborative study of the European Network of Teratology Information Services (ENTIS). *Reprod Toxicol*. 1996;10(4): 285–94.

McKenna K, Einarson A, Levinson A, Gideon K. Significant changes in antipsychotic drug use during pregnancy. *Vet Hum Toxicol*. 2004;46(1):44–6.

Menegola E, Broccia ML, Di Renzo F, Giavini E. Comparative study of sodium valproate–induced skeletal malformations using single or double staining methods. *Reprod Toxicol*. 2002;16(6):815–23.

Mhanna MJ, Bennet JB 2nd, Izatt SD. Potential fluoxetine chloride (Prozac) toxicity in a newborn. *Pediatrics*. 1997;100(1):158–9.

Misri S, Burgmann A, Kostaras D. Are SSRIs safe for pregnant and breast-feeding women? *Can Fam Physician*. 2000;46:626–8, 631–3.

Misri S, Carter D, Ryan D, Reebye P, Milis L. The clinical course of mood and anxiety disorders in pregnancy to 8 months postpartum: prospective cohort of 36 women. November 2005. Poster presented at the Canadian Psychiatric Association meeting.

Misri S, Milis L. Obsessive compulsive disorder in the postpartum: Open-label Quetiapine augmentation. *J. Clinical Psycho-pharmacology* 2004;24(6) 624–7.

Misri S, Oberlander TF, Fairbrother N, Carter D, Ryan D, Kuan AJ, Reebye P. Relation between prenatal maternal mood and anxiety and neonatal health. *Can J Psychiatry*. 2004;49(10):684–9.

Misri S, Reebye P, Oberlander TF, Carter D, Ryan D, Kendrick K. Internalizing behaviors of five-year-old children prenatally exposed to psychotropic medications. May 2005. Poster presented at the American Psychiatric Association meeting.

Montgomery SA, Henry J, McDonald G, Dinan T, Lader M, Hindmarch I, Clare A, Nutt D. Selective serotonin reuptake inhibitors: meta-analysis of discontinuation rates. *Int Clin Psychopharmacol*. 1994;9(1):47–53.

Montouris G. Gabapentin exposure in human pregnancy: results from the Gabapentin Pregnancy Registry. *Epilepsy Behav*. 2003;4(3):310–7.

Morag I, Batash D, Keidar R, Bulkowstein M, Heyman E. Paroxetine use throughout pregnancy: does it pose any risk to the neonate? *J Toxicol Clin Toxicol*. 2004;42(1):97–100.

Morrison JL, Chien C, Riggs KW, Gruber N, Rurak D. Effect of maternal fluoxetine administration on uterine blood flow, fetal blood gas status, and growth. *Pediatr Res*. 2002;51(4):433–42.

Mortensen JT, Olsen J, Larsen H, Bendsen J, Obel C, Sorensen HT. Psychomotor development in children exposed in utero to benzodiazepines, antidepressants, neuroleptics, and anti-epileptics. *Eur J Epidemiol*. 2003;18(8):769–71.

Nau H, Kuhnz W, Egger HJ, Rating D, Helge H. Anticonvulsants during pregnancy and lactation. Transplacental, maternal and neonatal pharmacokinetics. *Clin Pharmacokinet*. 1982;7(6):508–43.

Newport DJ, Hostetter A, Arnold A, Stowe ZN. The treatment of postpartum depression: minimizing infant exposures. *J Clin Psychiatry*. 2002;63 Suppl 7:31–44.

Nishiwaki T, Tanaka K, Sekiya S. Acute lithium intoxication in pregnancy. *Int J Gynaecol Obstet*. 1996;52(2):191–2.

Nonacs R, Cohen LS. Postpartum mood disorders: diagnosis and treatment guidelines. *J Clin Psychiatry*. 1998;59 Suppl 2:34–40.

Nonacs R, Cohen LS. Depression during pregnancy: diagnosis and treatment options. *J Clin Psychiatry*. 2002;63 Suppl 7:24–30.

Nordeng H, Lindemann R, Perminov KV, Reikvam A. Neonatal withdrawal syndrome after in utero exposure to selective serotonin reuptake inhibitors. *Acta Paediatr*. 2001;90(3):288–91.

Nulman I, Koren G. The safety of fluoxetine during pregnancy and lactation. *Teratology*. 1996;53(5):304–8.

Nulman I, Laslo D, Koren G. Treatment of epilepsy in pregnancy. *Drugs*. 1999; 57(4):535–44.

Nulman I, Rovet J, Stewart DE, Wolpin J, Gardner HA, Theis JG, Kulin N, Koren G. Neurodevelopment of children exposed in utero to antidepressant drugs. N Engl J Med. 1997;336(4):258–62.

Nulman I, Rovet J, Stewart DE, Wolpin J, Pace-Asciak P, Shuhaiber S, Koren G. Child development following exposure to tricyclic antidepressants or fluoxetine throughout fetal life: a prospective, controlled study. Am J Psychiatry. 2002;159(11):1389–95.

Oberlander TF, Eckstein Grunau R, Fitzgerald C, Ellwood AL, Misri S, Rurak D, Riggs KW. Prolonged prenatal psychotropic medication exposure alters neonatal acute pain response. Pediatr Res. 2002;51(4):443–53.

Oberlander TF, Grunau RE, Whitfield MF, Fitzgerald C, Pitfield S, Saul JP. Biobehavioral pain responses in former extremely low birth weight infants at four months' corrected age. Pediatrics. 2000;105(1):e6.

Oberlander TF, Misri S, Fitzgerald CE, Kostaras X, Rurak D, Riggs W. Pharmacologic factors associated with transient neonatal symptoms following prenatal psychotropic medication exposure. J Clin Psychiatry. 2004;65(2):230–7.

Ormond K, Pergament E. Update: benzodiazepines in pregnancy 7(4). Retrieved December 23, 2004, from http://www.fetal-exposure.org/BENZOUPDATE. html.

Pastuszak A, Schick-Boschetto B, Zuber C, Feldkamp M, Pinelli M, Sihn S, Donnenfeld A, McCormack M, Leen-Mitchell M, Woodland C, et al. Pregnancy outcome following first-trimester exposure to fluoxetine (Prozac). JAMA. 1993;269(17):2246–8.

Patton SW, Misri S, Corral MR, Perry KF, Kuan AJ. Antipsychotic medication during pregnancy and lactation in women with schizophrenia: evaluating the risk. Can J Psychiatry. 2002;47(10):959–65.

Pennell PB. The importance of monotherapy in pregnancy. Neurology. 2003;60(11 Suppl 4):S31–8.

Pennell PB. Antiepileptic drug pharmacokinetics during pregnancy and lactation. Neurology. 2003;61(6 Suppl 2):S35–42.

Pinelli JM, Symington AJ, Cunningham KA, Paes BA. Case report and review of the perinatal implications of maternal lithium use. Am J Obstet Gynecol. 2002;187(1):245–9.

Potvin W, Evans MF. Outcome of pregnancy following mothers' use of new SSRIs. Can Fam Physician. 1999;45:1477–9.

PsychNet. Compliance: improving patient adherence to antidepressant therapy. Mississauga: The Medicine Group Ltd, 1998.

Rampono J, Proud S, Hackett LP, Kristensen JH, Ilett KF. A pilot study of newer antidepressant concentrations in cord and maternal serum and possible effects in the neonate. Int J Neuropsychopharmacol. 2004:1–6.

Rasgon NL, Altshuler LL, Fairbanks L. Estrogen-replacement therapy for depression. *Am J Psychiatry.* 2001;158(10):1738.

Ratnayake T, Libretto SE. No complications with risperidone treatment before and throughout pregnancy and during the nursing period. *J Clin Psychiatry.* 2002;63(1):76–7.

Rayburn WF, Gonzalez CL, Parker KM, Christensen HD. Chronic prenatal exposure to carbamazepine and behavior effects on mice offspring. *Am J Obstet Gynecol.* 2004;190(2):517–21.

Rifkin A. Lithium discontinuation during pregnancy. *Am J Psychiatry.* 2001; 158(10):1741–2.

Robinson GE. Women and psychopharmacology. *Medscape Women's Health eJournal.* 2002;7(1).

Rohde A, Dembinski J, Dorn C. Mirtazapine (Remergil) for treatment resistant hyperemesis gravidarum: rescue of a twin pregnancy. *Arch Gynecol Obstet.* 2003;268:219–21.

Saks BR. Mirtazapine: treatment of depression, anxiety, hyperemesis gravidarum in the pregnant patient. A report of 7 cases. *Arch Womens Ment. Health.* 2001;3:165–70.

Samren EB, van Duijn CM, Christiaens GC, Hofman A, Lindhout D. Anti-epileptic drug regimens and major congenital abnormalities in the offspring. *Ann Neurol.* 1999;46(5):739–46.

Schou M. What happened later to the lithium babies? A follow-up study of children born without malformations. *Acta Psychiatr Scand.* 1976;54(3):193–7.

Schou M, Amdisen A. Lithium in pregnancy. *Lancet.* 1970;1(7661):1391.

Schou M, Amdisen A, Steenstrup OR. Lithium and pregnancy. II. Hazards to women given lithium during pregnancy and delivery. *Br Med J.* 1973; 2(5859):137–8.

Sichel DA, Cohen LS, Robertson LM, Ruttenberg A, Rosenbaum JF. Prophylactic estrogen in recurrent postpartum affective disorder. *Biol Psychiatry.* 1995;38(12):814–8.

Simhandl C, Zhoglami A, Pinder R. Pregnancy during use of mirtazapine. *Abstracts of the 21st C.I.N.P. Congress.* Glasgow, 1998.

Simon GE, Cunningham ML, Davis RL. Outcomes of prenatal antidepressant exposure. *Am J Psychiatry.* 2002;159(12):2055–61.

Smith MV, Rosenheck RA, Cavaleri MA, Howell HB, Poschman K, Yonkers KA. Screening for and detection of depression, panic disorder, and PTSD in public-sector obstetric clinics. *Psychiatr Serv.* 2004;55(4):407–14.

Soares CN, Viguera AC, Cohen L. Mood disturbance and pregnancy: pros and cons of pharmacologic treatment. *Rev Bras Psiquiatr.* 2001;23(1).

Steiner M. Perinatal mood disorders: position paper. *Psychopharmacol Bull.* 1998;34(3):301–6.

Stewart DE, Klompenhouwer JL, Kendell RE, van Hulst AM. Prophylactic lithium in puerperal psychosis. The experience of three centres. Br J Psychiatry. 1991;158:393–7.

Stingl J, Berghofer A, Bolk-Weischedel D. Healthy outcome and serum concentrations under olanzapine treatment in pregnant women. Clin Pharmacol Ther. 2000;67(2):129.

Stiskal JA, Kulin N, Koren G, Ho T, Ito S. Neonatal paroxetine withdrawal syndrome. Arch Dis Child Fetal Neonatal Ed. 2001;84(2):F134–5.

Stoner SC, Sommi RW, Jr., Marken PA, Anya I, Vaughn J. Clozapine use in two full-term pregnancies. J Clin Psychiatry. 1997;58(8):364–5.

Suri R, Burt VK, Altshuler LL, Zuckerbrow-Miller J, Fairbanks L. Fluvoxamine for postpartum depression. Am J Psychiatry. 2001;158(10):1739–40.

Sutherland JE, Sutherland SJ, Hoehns JD. Achieving the best outcome in treatment of depression. J Fam Pract. 2003;52(3):201–9.

Taylor TM, O'Toole MS, Ohlsen RI, Walters J, Pilowsky LS. Safety of quetiapine during pregnancy. Am J Psychiatry. 2003;160(3):588–9.

Tennis P, Eldridge RR. Preliminary results on pregnancy outcomes in women using lamotrigine. Epilepsia. 2002;43(10):1161–7.

Tenyi T, Trixler M, Keresztes Z. Quetiapine and pregnancy. Am J Psychiatry. 2002;159(4):674.

Tran TA, Leppik IE, Blesi K, Sathanandan ST, Remmel R. Lamotrigine clearance during pregnancy. Neurology. 2002;59(2):251–5.

Trindade E, Menon D, Topfer L-A, Coloma C. Adverse effects associated with selective serotonin reuptake inhibitors and tricyclic antidepressants: a meta-analysis. CMAJ 1998;159(10):1245–52.

Walker A, Rosenberg M, Balaban-Gil K. Neurodevelopmental and neurobehavioral sequelae of selected substances of abuse and psychiatric medications in utero. Child Adolesc Psychiatr Clin N Am. 1999;8(4):845–67.

Ward RK, Zamorski MA. Benefits and risks of psychiatric medications during pregnancy. Am Fam Physician. 2002;66(4):629–36.

Weinstock L, Cohen LS, Bailey JW, Blatman R, Rosenbaum JF. Obstetrical and neonatal outcome following clonazepam use during pregnancy: a case series. Psychother Psychosom. 2001;70(3):158–62.

Whooley MA, Simon GE. Managing depression in medical outpatients. N Engl J Med. 2000;343(26):1942–50.

Wide K, Winbladh B, Kallen B. Major malformations in infants exposed to antiepileptic drugs in utero, with emphasis on carbamazepine and valproic acid: a nation-wide, population-based register study. Acta Paediatr. 2004; 93(2):174–6.

Wisner KL, Gelenberg AJ, Leonard H, Zarin D, Frank E. Pharmacologic treatment of depression during pregnancy. JAMA. 1999;282(13):1264–9.

Wisner KL, Peindl KS, Gigliotti TV. Tricyclics vs SSRIs for postpartum depression. *Arch Womens Ment. Health*. 1999;1:189–91.

Wisner KL, Perel JM, Wheeler SB. Tricyclic dose requirements across pregnancy. *Am J Psychiatry*. 1993;150(10):1541–2.

Wisner KL, Zarin DA, Holmboe ES, Appelbaum PS, Gelenberg AJ, Leonard HL, Frank E. Risk-benefit decision making for treatment of depression during pregnancy. *Am J Psychiatry*. 2000;157(12):1933–40.

Yerby MS. The use of anticonvulsants during pregnancy. *Semin Perinatol*. 2001;25(3):153–8.

Yogev Y, Ben-Haroush A, Kaplan B. Maternal clozapine treatment and decreased fetal heart rate variability. *Int J Gynaecol Obstet*. 2002;79(3):259–60.

Yonkers KA, Wisner KL, Stowe Z, Leibenluft E, Cohen L, Miller L, Manber R, Viguera A, Suppes T, Altshuler L. Management of bipolar disorder during pregnancy and the postpartum period. *Am J Psychiatry*. 2004;161(4): 608–20.

Zeskind PS, Stephens LE. Maternal selective serotonin reuptake inhibitor use during pregnancy and newborn neurobehavior. *Pediatrics*. 2004;113(2): 368–75.

Chapter 9

American Academy of Pediatrics. The transfer of drugs and other chemicals into human milk. *Pediatrics*. 1994;93(1):137–50.

American Academy of Pediatrics. Work Group on Breast-feeding: breast-feeding and the use of human milk. *Pediatrics*. 1997;100:1035–9.

American Academy of Pediatrics. Transfer of drugs and other chemicals into human milk. *Pediatrics*. 2001;108(3):776–89.

Altshuler LL, Burt VK, McMullen M, Hendrick V. Breast-feeding and sertraline: a 24-hour analysis. *J Clin Psychiatry*. 1995;56(6):243–5.

Arnold LM, Suckow RF, Lichtenstein PK. Fluvoxamine concentrations in breast milk and in maternal and infant sera. *J Clin Psychopharmacol*. 2000; 20(4):491–3.

Austin MP, Mitchell PB. Use of psychotropic medications in breast-feeding women: acute and prophylactic treatment. *Aust NZ J Psychiatry*. 1998; 32(6):778–84.

Baab SW, Peindl KS, Piontek CM, Wisner KL. Serum bupropion levels in 2 breast-feeding mother-infant pairs. *J Clin Psychiatry*. 2002;63(10):910–1.

Bar-Oz B, Nulman I, Koren G, Ito S. Anticonvulsants and breast-feeding: a critical review. *Paediatr Drugs*. 2000;2(2):113–26.

Baum AL, Misri S. Selective serotonin-reuptake inhibitors in pregnancy and lactation. *Harv Rev Psychiatry*. 1996;4(3):117–25.

Begg EJ, Duffull SB, Saunders DA, Buttimore RC, Ilett KF, Hackett LP, Yapp P, Wilson DA. Paroxetine in human milk. *Br J Clin Pharmacol*. 1999;48(2): 142–7.

Berle JO, Steen VM, Aamo TO, Breilid H, Zahlsen K, Spigset O. Breast-feeding during maternal antidepressant treatment with serotonin reuptake inhibitors: infant exposure, clinical symptoms, and cytochrome P450 genotypes. *J Clin Psychiatry*. 2004;65:1228–34.

Birnbaum CS, Cohen LS, Bailey JW, Grush LR, Robertson LM, Stowe ZN. Serum concentrations of antidepressants and benzodiazepines in nursing infants: a case series. *Pediatrics*. 1999;104(1):e11.

Brent NB, Wisner KL. Fluoxetine and carbamazepine concentrations in a nursing mother/infant pair. *Clin Pediatr (Phila)*. 1998;37(1):41–4.

Breyer-Pfaff U, Nill K, Entenmann KN, Gaertner HJ. Secretion of amitriptyline and metabolites into breast milk. *Am J Psychiatry*. 1995;152(5):812–3.

Briggs GG, Samson JH, Ambrose PJ, Schroeder DH. Excretion of bupropion in breast milk. *Ann Pharmacother*. 1993;27(4):431–3.

Buist A. Treating mental illness in lactating women. *Medscape Womens Health*. 2001;6(2):3.

Buist A, Norman TR, Dennerstein L. Breast-feeding and the use of psychotropic medication: a review. *J Affect Disord*. 1990;19(3):197–206.

Burch KJ, Wells BG. Fluoxetine/norfluoxetine concentrations in human milk. *Pediatrics*. 1992;89(4 Pt 1):676–7.

Burt VK, Suri R, Altshuler L, Stowe Z, Hendrick VC, Muntean E. The use of psychotropic medications during breast-feeding. *Am J Psychiatry*. 2001; 158(7):1001–9.

Campagne D. Comment on "The effectiveness of various postpartum depression treatments and the impact of antidepressant drugs on nursing infants." *Medscape General Medicine*. 2004;6(1).

Chambers CD, Anderson FO, Thomas RG, Dick LM, Felix RJ, Johnson KA, Jones KL. Weight gain in infants breast-fed by mothers who take fluoxetine. *Pediatrics*. 1999;104(5):e61.

Chaudron LH, Jefferson JW. Mood stabilizers during breast-feeding: a review. *J Clin Psychiatry*. 2000;61(2):79–90.

Cohen LS, Viguera AC, Bouffard SM, Nonacs RM, Morabito C, Collins MH, Ablon JS. Venlafaxine in the treatment of postpartum depression. *J Clin Psychiatry*. 2001;62(8):592–6.

Croke S, Buist A, Hackett LP, Ilett KF, Norman TR, Burrows GD. Olanzapine excretion in human breast milk: estimation of infant exposure. *Int J Neuropsychopharmacol*. 2002;5(3):243–7.

Dahl ML, Olhager E, Ahlner J. Paroxetine withdrawal syndrome in a neonate. *Br J Psychiatry*. 1997;171:391–2.

Dharamsi A, Smith J. *Drugs in breast milk*. Vancouver, B.C.: British Columbia's Children's and Women's Pharmacy, Therapeutics and Nutrition Committee, 2003.

Dodd S, Maguire KP, Burrows GD, Norman TR. Nefazodone in the breast milk of nursing mothers: a report of two patients. *J Clin Psychopharmacol*. 2000;20(6):717–8.

Dodd S, Stocky A, Buist A, Burrows GD, Maguire K, Norman TR. Sertraline in paired blood plasma and breast-milk samples from nursing mothers. *Hum Psychopharmacol*. 2000;15(4):161–264.

Epperson N, Czarkowski KA, Ward-O'Brien D, Weiss E, Gueorguieva R, Jatlow P, Anderson GM. Maternal sertraline treatment and serotonin transport in breast-feeding mother-infant pairs. *Am J Psychiatry*. 2001;158 (10):1631–7.

Foglia JP, Sorisio D, Kirshner M, Pollock BG. Quantitative determination of paroxetine in plasma by high-performance liquid chromatography and ultraviolet detection. *J Chromatogr B Biomed Sci Appl*. 1997;693(1):147–51.

Frey OR, Scheidt P, von Brenndorff AI. Adverse effects in a newborn infant breast-fed by a mother treated with doxepin. *Ann Pharmacother*. 1999; 33(6):690–3.

Gjerdingen D. The effectiveness of various postpartum depression treatments and the impact of antidepressant drugs on nursing infants. *J Am Board Fam Pract*. 2003;16(5):372–82.

Goldstein DJ, Corbin LA, Fung MC. Olanzapine-exposed pregnancies and lactation: early experience. *J Clin Psychopharmacol*. 2000;20(4):399–403.

Hagg S, Granberg K, Carleborg L. Excretion of fluvoxamine into breast milk. *Br J Clin Pharmacol*. 2000;49(3):286–8.

Heikkinen T, Ekblad U, Kero P, Ekblad S, Laine K. Citalopram in pregnancy and lactation. *Clin Pharmacol Ther*. 2002;72(2):184–91.

Heikkinen T, Ekblad U, Laine K. Transplacental transfer of amitriptyline and nortriptyline in isolated perfused human placenta. *Psychopharmacology (Berl)*. 2001;153(4):450–4.

Heikkinen T, Ekblad U, Palo P, Laine K. Pharmacokinetics of fluoxetine and norfluoxetine in pregnancy and lactation. *Clin Pharmacol Ther*. 2003;73(4): 330–7.

Hendrick V, Altshuler L, Wertheimer A, Dunn WA. Venlafaxine and breast-feeding. *Am J Psychiatry*. 2001;158(12):2089–90.

Hendrick V, Fukuchi A, Altshuler L, Widawski M, Wertheimer A, Brunhuber MV. Use of sertraline, paroxetine and fluvoxamine by nursing women. *Br J Psychiatry*. 2001;179:163–6.

Hendrick V, Stowe ZN, Altshuler LL, Mintz J, Hwang S, Hostetter A, Suri R,

Leight K, Fukuchi A. Fluoxetine and norfluoxetine concentrations in nursing infants and breast milk. *Biol Psychiatry*. 2001;50(10):775–82.

Hill RC, McIvor RJ, Wojnar-Horton RE, Hackett LP, Ilett KF. Risperidone distribution and excretion into human milk: case report and estimated infant exposure during breast-feeding. *J Clin Psychopharmacol*. 2000;20(2):285–6.

Holmes LB, Harvey EA, Coull BA, Huntington KB, Khoshbin S, Hayes AM, Ryan LM. The teratogenicity of anticonvulsant drugs. *N Engl J Med*. 2001; 344(15):1132–8.

Holland D. An observation of the effect of sertraline on breast milk supply. *Aust NZ J Psychiatry*. 2000;34(6):1032.

Hostetter AL, Stowe ZN, Cox M, Ritchie JC. A novel system for the determination of antidepressant concentrations in human breast milk. *Ther Drug Monit*. 2004;26(1):47–52.

Ilett KF, Hackett LP, Dusci LJ, Roberts MJ, Kristensen JH, Paech M, Groves A, Yapp P. Distribution and excretion of venlafaxine and O-desmethylvenlafaxine in human milk. *Br J Clin Pharmacol*. 1998;45 (5):459–62.

Ilett KF, Hackett LP, Kristensen JH, Vaddadi KS, Gardiner SJ, Begg EJ. Transfer of risperidone and 9-hydroxyrisperidone into human milk. *Ann Pharmacother*. 2004;38(2):273–6.

Ilett KF, Kristensen JH, Hackett LP, Paech M, Kohan R, Rampono J. Distribution of venlafaxine and its O-desmethyl metabolite in human milk and their effects in breast-fed infants. *Br J Clin Pharmacol*. 2002;53(1):17–22.

Isenberg KE. Excretion of fluoxetine in human breast milk. *J Clin Psychiatry*. 1990;51(4):169.

Ito S, Blajchman A, Stephenson M, Eliopoulos C, Koren G. Prospective follow-up of adverse reactions in breast-fed infants exposed to maternal medication. *Am J Obstet Gynecol*. 1993;168(5):1393–9.

Ito S, Koren G. Antidepressants and breast-feeding. *Am J Psychiatry*. 1997;154(8):1174.

Kaye CM, Haddock RE, Langley PF, Mellow G, Tasker TCG, Zussman BD, Greb WH. A review of the metabolism and pharmacokinetics of paroxetine in man. *Acta Psychiatr Scand Suppl*. 1989;350:60–75.

Kristensen JH, Hackett LP, Kohan R, Paech M, Ilett KF. The amount of fluvoxamine in milk is unlikely to be a cause of adverse effects in breast-fed infants. *J Hum Lact*. 2002;18(2):139–43.

Kristensen JH, Ilett KF, Dusci LJ, Hackett LP, Yapp P, Wojnar-Horton RE, Roberts MJ, Paech M. Distribution and excretion of sertraline and N-desmethylsertraline in human milk. *Br J Clin Pharmacol*. 1998;45(5): 453–7.

Kristensen JH, Ilett KF, Hackett LP, Yapp P, Paech M, Begg EJ. Distribution and excretion of fluoxetine and norfluoxetine in human milk. *Br J Clin Pharmacol*. 1999;48(4):521–7.

Lebedevs TH, Wojnar-Horton RE, Yapp P, Roberts MJ, Dusci LJ, Hackett LP, Ilett KF. Excretion of temazepam in breast milk. *Br J Clin Pharmacol*. 1992;33(2):204–6.

Lester BM, Cucca J, Andreozzi L, Flanagan P, Oh W. Possible association between fluoxetine hydrochloride and colic in an infant. *J Am Acad Child Adolesc Psychiatry*. 1993;32(6):1253–5.

Liporace J, Kao A, D'Abreu A. Concerns regarding lamotrigine and breastfeeding. *Epilepsy Behav*. 2004;5(1):102–5.

Llewellyn A, Stowe ZN. Psychotropic medications in lactation. *J Clin Psychiatry*. 1998;59 Suppl 2:41–52.

Logsdon MC, Wisner K, Hanusa BH, Phillips A. Role functioning and symptom remission in women with postpartum depression after antidepressant treatment. *Arch Psychiatr Nurs*. 2003;17(6):276–83.

Longhurst JG, Weiss E. Use of psychotropic medications during lactation. *Am J Psychiatry*. 1998;155(11):1643.

Mammen OK, Perel JM, Rudolph G, Foglia JP, Wheeler SB. Sertraline and norsertraline levels in three breast-fed infants. *J Clin Psychiatry*. 1997;58(3): 100–3.

Misri S, Kim J, Riggs KW, Kostaras X. Paroxetine levels in postpartum depressed women, breast milk, and infant serum. *J Clin Psychiatry*. 2000; 61(11):828–32.

Misri S, Lusskin S.I. Treatment of psychiatric disorders in lactating women 2005; In: *UpToDate*, Ed. B. D. Rose, Wellesley, MA, 2005.

Misri S, Reebye P, Corral M, Milis L. The use of paroxetine and cognitive-behavioral therapy in postpartum depression and anxiety: A randomized controlled trial. *J Clin Psychiatry*. 2004;65:1236–41.

Misri S, Reebye P, Kendrick K, Carter D, Ryan D, Grunau RE, Oberlander TF. Internalizing behaviors in four-year-old children following in utero exposure to psychotropic medications. *American Journal of Psychiatry*, 2005.

Misri S, Sinclair DA, Kuan AJ. Breast-feeding and postpartum depression: is there a relationship? *Can J Psychiatry*. 1997;42(10):1061–5.

Moretti ME, Koren G, Verjee Z, Ito S. Monitoring lithium in breast milk: an individualized approach for breast-feeding mothers. *Ther Drug Monit*. 2003;25(3):364–6.

Newport DJ, Wilcox MM, Stowe ZN. Antidepressants during pregnancy and lactation: defining exposure and treatment issues. *Semin Perinatol*. 2001; 25(3):177–90.

Ohman I, Vitols S, Luef G, Soderfeldt B, Tomson T. Topiramate kinetics during delivery, lactation, and in the neonate: preliminary observations. *Epilepsia.* 2002;43(10):1157–60.

Ohman I, Vitols S, Tomson T. Lamotrigine in pregnancy: pharmacokinetics during delivery, in the neonate, and during lactation. *Epilepsia.* 2000; 41(6):709–13.

Ohman R, Hagg S, Carleborg L, Spigset O. Excretion of paroxetine into breast milk. *J Clin Psychiatry.* 1999;60(8):519–23.

Piontek CM, Baab S, Peindl KS, Wisner KL. Serum valproate levels in 6 breast-feeding mother-infant pairs. *J Clin Psychiatry.* 2000;61(3):170–2.

Piontek CM, Wisner KL, Perel JM, Peindl KS. Serum fluvoxamine levels in breast-fed infants. *J Clin Psychiatry.* 2001;62(2):111–3.

Rampono J, Kristensen JH, Hackett LP, Paech M, Kohan R, Ilett KF. Citalopram and demethylcitalopram in human milk; distribution, excretion and effects in breast-fed infants. *Br J Clin Pharmacol.* 2000;50(3):263–8.

Schmidt K, Olesen OV, Jensen PN. Citalopram and breast-feeding: serum concentration and side effects in the infant. *Biol Psychiatry.* 2000;47(2):164–5.

Schou M, Amdisen A. Lithium and pregnancy. 3. Lithium ingestion by children breast-fed by women on lithium treatment. *Br Med J.* 1973;2(5859):138.

Spigset O, Corleborg L, Ohman R, Norstrom A. Excretion of citalopram in breast milk. *Br J Clin Pharmacol.* 1997;44(3):295–8.

Spigset O, Corleborg L, Norstrom A, Sandlund M. Paroxetine level in breast milk. *J Clin Psychiatry.* 1996;57(1):39.

Stowe ZN, Hostetter AL, Owens MJ, Ritchie JC, Sternberg K, Cohen LS, Nemeroff CB. The pharmacokinetics of sertraline excretion into human breast milk: determinants of infant serum concentrations. *J Clin Psychiatry.* 2003;64(1):73–80.

Stowe ZN, Cohen LS, Hostetter A, Ritchie JC, Owens MJ, Nemeroff CB. Paroxetine in human breast milk and nursing infants. *Am J Psychiatry.* 2000;157(2):185–9.

Stowe ZN, Strader JR, Nemeroff CB. Psychopharmacology during pregnancy and lactation. In: Schatzberg AF, Nemeroff CB (eds.). *The American Psychiatric Press textbook of psychopharmacology,* 2nd ed. Washington, DC: American Psychiatric Press, 1998.

Stowe ZN, Owens MJ, Landry JC, Kilts CD, Ely T, Llewellyn A, Nemeroff CB. Sertraline and desmethylsertraline in human breast milk and nursing infants. *Am J Psychiatry.* 1997;154(9):1255–60.

Suri R, Stowe ZN, Hendrick V, Hostetter A, Widawski M, Altshuler LL. Estimates of nursing infant daily dose of fluoxetine through breast milk. *Biol Psychiatry.* 2002;52(5):446–51.

Suri RA, Altshuler LL, Burt VK, Hendrick VC. Managing psychiatric medications in the breast-feeding woman. *Medscape Womens Health*. 1998;3(1):1.

Taddio A, Ito S, Koren G. Excretion of fluoxetine and its metabolite, norfluoxetine, in human breast milk. *J Clin Pharmacol*. 1996;36(1):42–7.

Tenyi T, Csabi G, Trixler M. Antipsychotics and breast-feeding: a review of the literature. *Paediatr Drugs*. 2000;2(1):23–8.

Weissman AM, Levy BT, Hartz AJ, Bentler S, Donohue M, Ellingrod VL, Wisner KL. Pooled analysis of antidepressant levels in lactating mothers, breast milk, and nursing infants. *Am J Psychiatry*. 2004;161:1066–78.

Whalley LJ, Blain PG, Prime JK. Haloperidol secreted in breast milk. *Br Med J (Clin Res Ed)*. 1981;282(6278):1746–7.

Winans EA. Antipsychotics and breast-feeding. *J Hum Lact*. 2001;17(4): 344–7.

Winans EA. Antidepressant use during lactation. *J Hum Lact*. 2001;17(3): 256–61.

Wisner KL, Findling RL, Perel JM. Paroxetine in breast milk. *Am J Psychiatry*. 2001;158(1):144–5.

Wisner KL, Perel JM. Serum levels of valproate and carbamazepine in breast-feeding mother-infant pairs. *J Clin Psychopharmacol*. 1998;18(2):167–9.

Wisner KL, Perel JM, Blumer J. Serum sertraline and N-desmethylsertraline levels in breast-feeding mother-infant pairs. *Am J Psychiatry*. 1998;155(5): 690–2.

Wisner KL, Perel JM, Findling RL. Antidepressant treatment during breast-feeding. *Am J Psychiatry*. 1996;153(9):1132–7.

Wisner KL, Perel JM, Findling RL, Hinnes RL. Nortriptyline and its hydroxy-metabolites in breast-feeding mothers and newborns. *Psychopharmacol Bull*. 1997;33(2):249–51.

Wisner KL, Perel JM, Foglia JP. Serum clomipramine and metabolite levels in four nursing mother-infant pairs. *J Clin Psychiatry*. 1995;56(1):17–20.

Wisner K, Perel J, Peindl K, Hanusa B, et al. Prevention of postpartum depression: a pilot randomized clinical trial. *Am J Psychiatry*. 2004;161:1290–92.

Wright S, Dawling S, Ashford JJ. Excretion of fluvoxamine in breast milk. *Br J Clin Pharmacol*. 1991;31(2):209.

Yonkers KA, Wisner KL, Stowe Z, Leibenluft E, Cohen L, Miller L, Manber R, Viguera A, Suppes T, Altshuler L. Management of bipolar disorder during pregnancy and the postpartum period. *Am J Psychiatry*. 2004;161(4):608–20.

Yoshida K, Smith B, Craggs M, Kumar RC. Investigation of pharmacokinetics and of possible adverse effects in infants exposed to tricyclic antidepressants in breast-milk. *J Affect Disord*. 1997;43(3):225–37.

Yoshida K, Smith B, Craggs M, Kumar RC. Fluoxetine in breast-milk and developmental outcome of breast-fed infants. *Br J Psychiatry*. 1998;172:175–8.

Yoshida K, Smith B, Kumar R. Psychotropic drugs in mothers' milk: a comprehensive review of assay methods, pharmacokinetics and of safety of breast-feeding. *J Psychopharmacol.* 1999;13(1):64–80.

Yoshida K, Smith B, Kumar RC. Fluvoxamine in breast-milk and infant development. *Br J Clin Pharmacol.* 1997;44(2):210–1.

Chapter 10

Appleby L, Hirst E, Marshall S, Keeling F, Brind J, Butterworth T, Lole J. The treatment of postnatal depression by health visitors: impact of brief training on skills and clinical practice. *J Affect Disord.* 2003;77(3):261–6.

Appleby L, Warner R, Whitton A, Faragher B. A controlled study of fluoxetine and cognitive-behavioural counselling in the treatment of postnatal depression. *BMJ.* 1997;314(7085):932–6.

Austin MP. Targeted group antenatal prevention of postnatal depression: a review. *Acta Psychiatr Scand.* 2003;107(4):244–50.

Boath E, Cox J, Lewis M, Jones P, Pryce A. When the cradle falls: the treatment of postnatal depression in a psychiatric day hospital compared with routine primary care. *J Affect Disord.* 1999;53(2):143–51.

Bowlby J. *Maternal care and mental health.* Monograph series no. 2. Geneva: World Health Organisation, 1951.

Brugha TS, Sharp HM, Cooper SA, Weisender C, Britto D, Shinkwin R, Sherrif T, Kirwan PH. The Leicester 500 Project. Social support and the development of postnatal depressive symptoms, a prospective cohort survey. *Psychol Med.* 1998;28(1):63–79.

Chabrol H, Teissedre F, Saint-Jean M, Teisseyre N, Roge B, Mullet E. Prevention and treatment of post-partum depression: a controlled randomized study on women at risk. *Psychol Med.* 2002;32(6):1039–47.

Corral M, Kuan A, Kostaras D. Bright light therapy's effect on postpartum depression. *Am J Psychiatry.* 2000;157(2):303–4.

Cunningham M, Zayas LH. Reducing depression in pregnancy: designing multimodal interventions. *Soc Work.* 2002;47(2):114–23.

Elliott SA, Leverton TJ, Sanjack M, Turner H, Cowmeadow P, Hopkins J, Bushnell D. Promoting mental health after childbirth: a controlled trial of primary prevention of postnatal depression. *Br J Clin Psychol.* 2000;39 (Pt 3):223–41.

Epperson CN, Terman M, Terman JS, Hanusa BH, Oren DA, Peindl KS, Wisner KL. Randomized clinical trial of bright light therapy for antepartum depression: preliminary findings. *J Clin Psychiatry.* 2004;65(3):421–5.

Field T, Grizzle N, Scafidi F, Abrams S, Richardson S. Massage therapy for infants of depressed mothers. *Infant Behav Dev.* 1996;19:107–12.

Fisher J, Feekery C, Rowe H. Treatment of maternal mood disorder and infant behaviour disturbance in an Australian private mothercraft unit: a follow-up study. *Arch Women Ment Health*. 2004;7(1):89–93.

Gorman JM. Medication and cognitive-behavioral therapy during pregnancy. *CNS Spectr*. 2004;9(3):170.

Hendrick V. Treatment of postnatal depression. *BMJ*. 2003;327(7422):1003–4.

Klier CM, Muzik M, Rosenblum KL, Lenz G. Interpersonal psychotherapy adapted for the group setting in the treatment of postpartum depression. *J Psychother Pract Res*. 2001;10(2):124–31.

Kumar R, Marks M, Platz C, Yoshida K. Clinical survey of a psychiatric mother and baby unit: characteristics of 100 consecutive admissions. *J Affect Disord*. 1995;33(1):11–22.

Linde K, Ramirez G, Mulrow CD, Pauls A, Weidenhammer W, Melchart D. St. John's wort for depression—an overview and meta-analysis of randomised clinical trials. *BMJ*. 1996;313(7052):253–8.

Logsdon MC, Birkimer JC, Usui WM. The link of social support and postpartum depressive symptoms in African-American women with low incomes. *MCN Am J Matern Child Nurs*. 2000;25(5):262–6.

Lumley J, Austin MP. What interventions may reduce postpartum depression. *Curr Opin Obstet Gynecol*. 2001;13(6):605–11.

MacArthur C, Winter HR, Bick DE, Knowles H, Lilford R, Henderson C, Lancashire RJ, Braunholtz DA, Gee H. Effects of redesigned community postnatal care on women's health 4 months after birth: a cluster randomised controlled trial. *Lancet*. 2002;359(9304):378–85.

Main T. Mothers and children in psychiatric hospital. *Lancet*. 1948;11: 1845.

Marangell LB, Martinez JM, Zboyan HA, Chong H, Puryear LJ. Omega-3 fatty acids for the prevention of postpartum depression: negative data from a preliminary, open-label pilot study. *Depress Anxiety*. 2004;19(1):20–3.

McGrath PJ, Elgar FJ, Johnston C, Dozois DJ, Reyno S. Treating maternal depression? *Br J Psychiatry*. 2003;183:461–2; author reply 462.

McVeigh CA. Investigating the relationship between satisfaction with social support and functional status after childbirth. *MCN Am J Matern Child Nurs*. 2000;25(1):25–30.

Meager I, Milgrom J. Group treatment for postpartum depression: a pilot study. *Aust N Z J Psychiatry*. 1996;30(6):852–60.

Milgrom J, Burrows GD, Snellen M, Stamboulakis W, Burrows K. Psychiatric illness in women: a review of the function of a specialist mother-baby unit. *Aust N Z J Psychiatry*. 1998;32(5):680–6.

Misri S, Reebye P, Corral M, et al. The use of paroxetine and cognitive-behavioral therapy in postpartum depression and anxiety: a randomized controlled trial. *J Clin Psychiatry* 2004;65:1236–41.

Morgan M, Matthey S, Barnett B, Richardson C. A group programme for post-natally distressed women and their partners. *J Adv Nurs.* 1997;26(5):913–20.

Morrell CJ, Spiby H, Stewart P, Walters S, Morgan A. Costs and effectiveness of community postnatal support workers: randomised controlled trial. *BMJ.* 2000;321(7261):593–8.

Murray L, Cooper PJ, Wilson A, Romaniuk H. Controlled trial of the short- and long-term effect of psychological treatment of post-partum depression: 2. Impact on the mother-child relationship and child outcome. *Br J Psychiatry.* 2003;182:420–7.

Ogrodniczuk JS, Piper WE. Preventing postnatal depression: a review of research findings. *Harv Rev Psychiatry.* 2003;11(6):291–307.

O'Hara MW, Stuart S, Gorman LL, Wenzel A. Efficacy of interpersonal psychotherapy for postpartum depression. *Arch Gen Psychiatry.* 2000;57(11):1039–45.

Oren DA, Wisner KL, Spinelli M, Epperson CN, Peindl KS, Terman JS, Terman M. An open trial of morning light therapy for treatment of antepartum depression. *Am J Psychiatry.* 2002;159(4):666–9.

Parry BL, Curran ML, Stuenkel CA, Yokimozo M, Tam L, Powell KA, Gillin JC. Can critically timed sleep deprivation be useful in pregnancy and postpartum depressions? *J Affect Disord.* 2000;60(3):201–12.

Robinson L, Walker JR, Anderson D. Cognitive-behavioural treatment of panic disorder during pregnancy and lactation. *Can J Psychiatry.* 1992;37(9):623–6.

Severus WE, Littman AB, Stoll AL. Omega-3 fatty acids, homocysteine, and the increased risk of cardiovascular mortality in major depressive disorder. *Harv Rev Psychiatry.* 2001;9(6):280–93.

Shelton RC, Keller MB, Gelenberg A, Dunner DL, Hirschfeld R, Thase ME, Russell J, Lydiard RB, Crits-Cristoph P, Gallop R, Todd L, Hellerstein D, Goodnick P, Keitner G, Stahl SM, Halbreich U. Effectiveness of St. John's wort in major depression: a randomized controlled trial. *JAMA.* 2001;285(15):1978–86.

Spinelli MG. Interpersonal psychotherapy for depressed antepartum women: a pilot study. *Am J Psychiatry.* 1997;154(7):1028–30.

Spinelli MG, Endicott J. Controlled clinical trial of interpersonal psychotherapy versus parenting education program for depressed pregnant women. *Am J Psychiatry.* 2003;160(3):555–62.

Stuart S, O'Hara MW. Interpersonal psychotherapy for postpartum depression. *J Psychother Pract Res.* 1995;4:18–29.

Stuart S, O'Hara MW, Gorman LL. The prevention and psychotherapeutic treatment of postpartum depression. *Arch Women Ment Health*. 2003;6 Suppl 2:S57–69.

Tam WH, Lee DT, Chiu HF, Ma KC, Lee A, Chung TK. A randomised controlled trial of educational counselling on the management of women who have suffered suboptimal outcomes in pregnancy. *BJOG*. 2003;110(9):853–9.

Tao D. Research on the reduction of anxiety and depression with acupuncture. *Am J Acupuncture*. 1993;21:327–9.

Webster J, Linnane J, Roberts J, Starrenburg S, Hinson J, Dibley L. IDentify, Educate and Alert (IDEA) trial: an intervention to reduce postnatal depression. *BJOG*. 2003;110(9):842–6.

Weier KM, Beal MW. Complementary therapies as adjuncts in the treatment of postpartum depression. *J Midwifery Womens Health*. 2004;49(2):96–104.

Zlotnick C, Johnson SL, Miller IW, Pearlstein T, Howard M. Postpartum depression in women receiving public assistance: pilot study of an interpersonal-therapy-oriented group intervention. *Am J Psychiatry*. 2001;158(4): 638–40.

Chapter 11

Barker DJP. Fetal origins of coronary heart disease. *BMJ*. 1995;311:171–4.

Bayley N. *Bayley scales of infant development*, 2nd ed. Orlando, FL: The Psychological Corporation, 1993.

Chung TKH, Lau TK, Yip ASK, Chiu HFK, Lee DTS. Antepartum depressive symptomatology is associated with adverse obstetric and neonatal outcomes. *Psychosomatic Medicine*. 2001;63:830–4.

Clarke AS, Wittwer DJ, Abbott DH, Schneider ML. Long-term effects of prenatal stress on HPA axis activity in juvenile rhesus monkeys. *Dev Psychobiol*. 1994;27:257–69.

Copher DE, Huber CP. Heart rate responses of the human fetus to induced maternal hypoxia. *Am J Obstet Gynecol*. 1967;98:320–35.

Copper RL, Goldenberg RL, Das A, Elder N, Swain M, Norman G, Ramsey R, Cotroneo P, Collins BA, Johnson F, et al. The preterm prediction study: maternal stress is associated with spontaneous preterm birth at less than 35 weeks' gestation. *Am J Obstet Gynecol*. 1996;175:1286–92.

Cranley MS. Development of a tool for the measurement of maternal attachment during pregnancy. *Nurs Res*. 1981;30:281–4.

DiPietro JA, Hodgson DM, Costigan KA, Hilton SC, Johnson TR. Fetal neurobehavioral development. *Child Dev*. 1996;67:2553–67.

Erickson K, Thorsen P, Chrousos G, Grigoriadis DE, Khongsaly O, McGregor J,

Schulkin J. Preterm birth: associated neuroendocrine, medical, and behavioral risk factors. *J Clin Endocrinol Metab*. 1987;64:1054–59.

Eskes TK. Obstetrical consequences of unresolved mourning over the death of an infant in the perinatal period. *Nederlands Tijdschrif voor Geneeskunde*. 1985;129:433–36.

Field T, Diego M, Hernandez-Reif M, Schanberg S, Kuhn C, Yando R, Bendell D. Pregnancy anxiety and comorbid depression and anger: effects on the fetus and neonate. *Depress Anxiety*. 2003;17:140–51.

Glover V. Maternal stress or anxiety during pregnancy and the development of the baby. *The Practicing Midwife*. 1999;2(5):20–2.

Groome LJ, Swiber MJ, Bentz LS, Holland SB, Atterbury JL. Maternal anxiety during pregnancy: effect on fetal behaviour at 38 to 40 weeks of gestation. *J Dev Behav Pediatr*. 1995;16:391–96.

Hobel CJ, Dunkel-Schetter C, Roesch SC, Castro LC, Arora CP. Maternal plasma corticotropin-releasing hormone associated with stress at 20 weeks' gestation in pregnancies ending in preterm delivery. *Am J Obstet Gynecol*. 1999;180:S257–63.

Holzman C, Jetton J, Siler-Khodr T, Fisher R, Rip T. Second trimester corticotropin-releasing hormone levels in relation to preterm delivery and ethnicity. *Obstet Gynecol*. 2001;97:657–63.

Institute of Medicine, National Academy of Sciences. *Preventing low birthweight*. Washington, DC: National Academy Press, 1985.

Leader LR, Correira IG. *Can television influence fetal behaviour?* Abstract presented at the 10th International Congress of the International Society of Prenatal and Perinatal Psychology and Medicine, Cracow, Poland, 1992.

Lindgren K. Relationships among maternal-fetal attachment, prenatal depression, and health practices in pregnancy. *Res Nurs Health*. 2001;24(3):203–17.

Lundy B, Field T, Pickens J. Newborns of mothers with depressive symptoms are less expressive. *Infant Behav Dev*. 1996;19:419–24.

Meier A. Child psychiatric sequelae of maternal war stress. *Acta Psychiatr Scand*. 1985;72:505–11.

Misri S, Oberlander T, Fairbrother N, Carter C, Ryan D, Kuan AJ, Reebye P. Relation between prenatal maternal mood and anxiety and neonatal health. *Can J Psychiatry*. 2004;49(10):684–9.

Omer H. Possible psychophysiologic mechanisms in premature labor. *Psychosomatics*. 1986;27:580–4.

Rondo PH, Ferreira RF, Nogueira F, Ribeiro MC, Lobert H, Artes R. Maternal psychological stress and distress as predictors of low birth weight, prematurity and intrauterine growth retardation. *Eur J Clin Nutr*. 2003;57(2):266–72.

Rowley DL, Hogue CJR, Blackmore CA, et al. Preterm delivery among African-

American women: a research strategy. In: Rowley D, Tosteson H, eds. *Racial differences in preterm delivery: developing a new research paradigm.* 1–6. New York: Oxford University Press, 1994.

Schneider ML, Roughton EC, Koehler AJ, Lubach GR. Growth development following prenatal stress exposure in primates: an examination of ontogenetic vulnerability. *Child Dev.* 1999;70:263–74.

Steer RA, Scholl TO, Hediger MI, Fischer RL. Self-reported depression and negative pregnancy outcomes. *J Clin Epidemiol.* 1992;45:1093–99.

Stokvis B. *Het verzien in de zwangerschap, medisch en psychologisch beschouwd.* Lochem: NV Uitgeversmaatschappij de Tijdstroom, 1940.

Teixeira JM, Fisk NM, Glover V. Association between maternal anxiety in pregnancy and increased uterine artery resistance index: cohort based study. *BMJ.* 1999;318(7177):153–7.

Van den Bergh BR. The influence of maternal emotions during pregnancy on fetal and neonatal behaviour. *J Prenat Perinat Psychol Med.* 1990;5:119–30.

Wadhwa PD, Porto M, Garite TJ, Chicz-DeMet A, Sandman, CA. Maternal corticotropin-releasing hormone levels in the early third trimester predict length of gestation in human pregnancy. *Am J Obstet Gynecol.* 1998;79:1079–85.

Wadhwa PD, Sandman CA, Porto M, Dunkel-Schetter C, Garite TJ. The association between prenatal stress and infant birth weight and gestational age at birth: a prospective investigation. *Am J Obstet Gynecol.* 1993;169:858–65.

Weinstock M, Matlina E, Maor GI, Rosen H, McEwen BS. Prenatal stress selectively alters the reactivity of the hypothalamic-pituitary adrenal system in the female rat. *Brain Res.* 1992;595:195–200.

Zuckerman B, Bauchner H, Parker S, Cabral H. Maternal depressive symptoms during pregnancy and newborn irritability. *J Dev Behav Pediatr.* 1990;11:190–4.

Chapter 12

Abramowitz J, Moore K, Carmin C, Wiegartz PS, Purdon C. Acute onset of obsessive-compulsive disorder in males following childbirth. *Psychosomatics.* 2001;42(5):429–31.

Abramowitz J, Schwartz S, Moore K. Obsessional thoughts in postpartum females and their partners: content, severity and relationship with depression. *J Clin Psychol Med Settings.* 2003;10(3):157–64.

Deater-Deckard K, Pickering K, Dunn JF, Golding J. Family structure and depressive symptoms in men preceding and following the birth of a child. The

Avon Longitudinal Study of Pregnancy and Childhood Study Team. *Am J Psychiatry.* 1998;155(6):818–23.

Goodman JH. Paternal postpartum depression, its relationship to maternal postpartum depression, and implications for family health. *J Adv Nurs.* 2004;45(1):26–35.

Kleiman K. *The postpartum husband: practical solutions for living with postpartum depression.* Philadelphia: Xlibris, 2000.

Klein H. Couvade syndrome: male counterpart to pregnancy. *Int J Psychiatry Med.* 1991;21(1):57–69.

Matthey S, Barnett B, Ungerer J, Waters B. Paternal and maternal depressed mood during the transition to parenthood. *J Affect Disord.* 2000;60(2):75–85.

Meighan M, Davis M, Thomas S, Droppleman P. Living with postpartum depression: the father's experience. *MCN Am J Matern Child Nurs.* 1999; 24(4):202.

Misri S, Kostaras X, Fox D, Kostaras D. The impact of partner support in the treatment of postpartum depression. *Can J Psychiatry.* 2000;45(6):554–8.

Tammentie T, Paavilainen E, Astedt-Kurki P, Tarkka MT. Family dynamics of postnatally depressed mothers—discrepancy between expectations and reality. *J Clin Nurs.* 2004;13(1):65–74.

INDEX

ABOUT THE AUTHOR

SHAILA KULKARNI MISRI, M.D., F.R.C.P.C., is one of the leading reproductive psychiatrists in North America and is internationally recognized as a pioneer in women's mental health and reproductive issues. She is the founder and director of Reproductive Mental Health at both St. Paul's Hospital and BC Women's Hospital & Health Centre in Vancouver, and Clinical Professor of Psychiatry and Obstetrics and Gynecology at the University of British Columbia, Canada.